The Dependence Phenomenon

The Dependence Phenomenon

Edited by

M. M. Glatt and J. Marks

MTP PRESS LIMITED
International Medical Publishers

Published by
MTP Press Limited
Falcon House
Lancaster, England

First published 1982

British Library Cataloguing in Publication Data
The Dependence phenomenon.
1. Drug abuse
I. Glatt, Max II. Marks, J.
616.86 RC564

ISBN 0-85200-414-1

Printed in Great Britain by
Butler & Tanner Ltd, Frome and London

Contents

List of Contributors

M. M. GLATT
Jellinek Unit,
The Charter Clinic,
Radnor Walk
London SW3 9PB

W. KEUP
J. Schauer-Strasse 16
D-8039 Puchheim/Munchen
West Germany

J. H. LACEY
St George's Hospital
Cranmer Terrace
London SW17, UK

J. H. LANGER
Preventive Programs Section
Office of Public Affairs, Drug Enforcement Administration
US Department of Justice
DC 20537 USA

J. W. LEWIS
Pharmaceutical Division
Reckitt and Colman
Dansom Lane
Kingston-upon-Hull
Humberside, UK

J. MARKS
Girton College
Cambridge, UK

M. RAW
Psychology Department
St George's Hospital Medical School
Cranmer Terrace
London SW17, UK

H. B. SPEAR
Home Office
Queen Anne's Gate
London SW1, UK

F. WELLS
British Medical Association
Tavistock House
Tavistock Square
London WC1, UK

Foreword

... there is scarcely any agent which can be taken into the body to which some individuals will not get a reaction satisfactory or pleasurable to them, persuading them to continue its use even to the point of abuse ...

Eddy (1965)

Dependence is one of the major problems of our modern society both in industrialized and developing nations. There is, however, nothing new in man's dependence on drugs.

For many centuries past, there can be few people throughout the world who do not 'overuse', 'misuse' or 'abuse' some drugs. For many the drugs that are 'overused' are caffeine (from tea or coffee), nicotine (from tobacco) or alcohol (from beer, wine or spirits), all socially accepted normal ingredients of everyday life in most communities. For a smaller group 'misuse' concerns commonly prescribed medical substances, such as barbiturates, amphetamines. For an even smaller group there is the less socially acceptable 'abuse' of specific drugs such as morphine and related analgesics, cannabis, or hallucinogens.

Man has employed such drugs in an attempt to banish pain and discomfort, to attain a state of oblivion, or alternatively, euphoria or ecstasy, or to escape from unpleasant reality into a much more agreeable state of fantasy. From time to time some drug may have been regarded as sacred by one culture, but condemned as a devil's instrument by another. Over the ages many such drugs that affect the mind have gained and lost popularity. Some of the best known among them – such as alcohol, the opiates and cannabis, so popular in many parts of the world today – have been great favourites for thousands of years even though their popularity waxed and waned and varied from culture to culture.

Much of this field of study is still covered with confusion, not only because the socially acceptable practices of one generation or community are the legally enforceable abuses of another, but because much of the terminology employed has become subject to lack of general agreement.

The Dependence Phenomenon

Drug dependence, according to the 1969 World Health Organization definition (WHO, 1969), is

> a state, psychic and sometimes also physical, resulting from the interaction between a living organism and a drug, characterised by behavioural and other responses that always include a compulsion to take the drug on a continuous or periodic basis in order to experience its psychic effects, and sometimes to avoid the discomfort of its absence. Tolerance may or may not be present. A person may be dependent on more than one drug

and polydrug misuse is nowadays more common in some western countries than the use of just one drug.

It is interesting to note that the current definition refers to 'compulsion' to take the drug, while the older and revised form (WHO, 1957) expanded this to include also an 'overpowering desire' or need. Drug misusers and uncontrolled drinkers often used the alternative term 'overwhelming'. But these terms merely denote a relative and not an absolute state. What is experienced as absolutely overpowering and overwhelming by one individual, in a given situation and under certain circumstances, can be tolerated with a major or minor effort by another individual possibly under a somewhat different set of circumstances. In all aspects of drug dependence not only the 'agent' (the pharmacological nature of the drug concerned) but also the psychological biological makeup of an individual ('host') and social and other environmental factors always have to be considered (Glatt, 1974). This applies to aetiology, the pace of developmental progress of the dependence, treatment, rehabilitation, prevention, prognosis etc. and is reflected in this volume. All too often in the past attention was mainly directed to the nature of the drug without considering the drug user's personality and his social environment.

Dependence can be psychological and/or physical. Contrary to popular belief it is psychological dependence and not physical dependence which in the long run constitutes the main problem. Physical abstinence syndromes can be very distressing and even life-threatening, but with skilled supervision, this acute withdrawal syndrome can usually be handled relatively easily. But psychological dependence is what makes drug dependence so difficult to deal with in the long run, and is responsible for the unfortunate fact that, essentially, states of drug dependence are relapsing disorders. Social factors, too, such as 'subcultures', peer pressure, social conditioning etc. may play a role in precipitating a relapse, after the individual had experienced a period of freedom from drug use.

The current concept of dependence on substances obviously includes both legally used and often widely socially accepted drugs, such as alcohol and tobacco, as well as illicit drugs. The fact that some drugs are legal and others illicit does not in itself tell us anything about the risks or otherwise attached to their use or misuse. Likewise the fact that such a drug or substance has been traditionally accepted by society, whether it is alcohol, tobacco, or even coffee and tea, or prescribed by the doctor, does not provide a guarantee or an immunity against the development of a state of more or less dangerous dependency. In most countries the problem caused by misuse of, and dependence upon, legal drugs, in particular alcohol, are much more widespread than those posed by illicit drugs; and in many countries the overprescribing and overconsumption of pharmaceuticals also constitutes a significant problem.

Dependence is a complex phenomenon that, as we have seen, may vary in its manifestations according to social environment, local fashion and subculture, regional or national characteristics etc. Cultural acceptance of a given substance or otherwise may even affect symptomatology and the type of personality predominant among drug misusers as reflected, for example, in the difference between the predominantly sociogenic French delta alcoholic (not particularly plagued by guilt feelings over his drinking) and the often sociogenic Anglo-American gamma alcoholic (with his acute, overwhelming remorse the morning after).

Both of us have stressed in the past (Glatt, 1978; Marks, 1978) that dependence should be regarded in a wider context to include, for example, gambling. One of us (Marks, 1978) has pressed the argument further and spoken about a 'spectrum of dependence'. On this basis it is argued that for a broad-range of human activities that produce a mood change, dependence can occur if this is measured in terms of an unnatural drive towards the specific pleasure-seeking goal. Within these pleasure-giving activities the question of social acceptability is based merely on a value judgement. Such a judgement is difficult, for there are no scientifically definable borders or limits between the various grades of dependence that exist. It was argued that we should view the whole range of pleasure-giving activities as a spectrum (Figure 1). At one end of the scale are the universal commonplace enjoyments to which no one can object, at the other the socially unacceptable patterns of those dependent, for example, on heroin. Between these extremes are dependencies for which we can assign a rating biased by social fashion or our culture, nation and age and by our own predelictions and aversions. Even with an accepted rating order, it is difficult to define the borders between acceptability and non-acceptability without value judgements that are subject to bias.

This view has been criticized Smith (1980) and is not accepted as a valid concept by Keup in this book (Chapter 1). Stepney (1980) on the other hand has propounded a similar model for pleasure-giving 'habits', one class of which includes substances of dependence. In an area where knowledge is negligible, such controversy is good, particularly if it encourages further thought and experiment.

For this book we have deliberately chosen the provocative title of 'The Dependence Phenomenon' and accepted a broad interpretation of the term dependence. While it touches on many aspects of the subject of dependence this present volume does not attempt to cover the whole subject comprehensively and systematically. Rather does it aim at discussing in greater depth some of the key issues of the subject today.

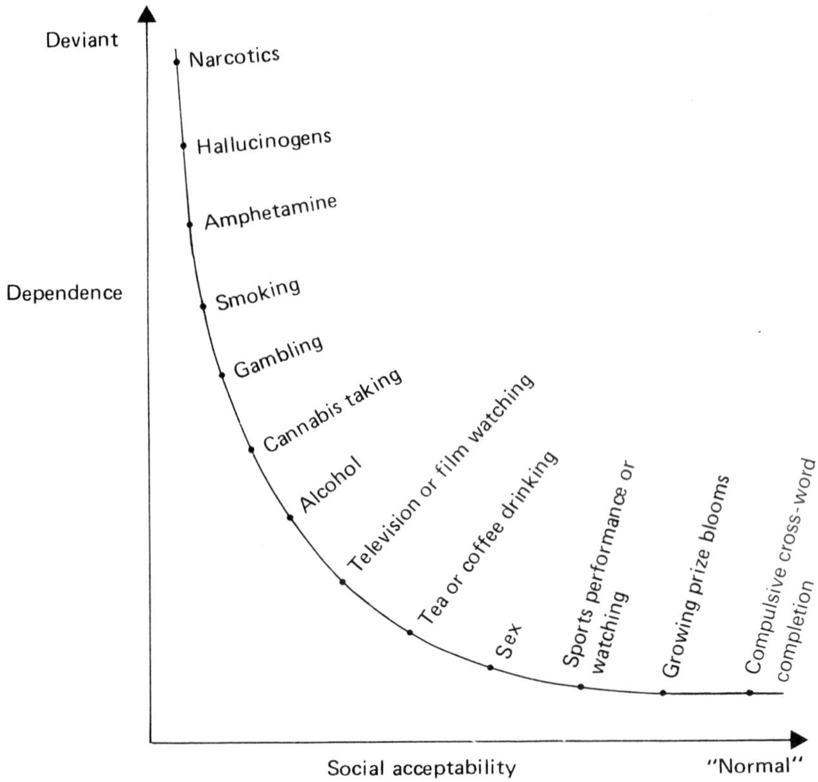

Figure 1 The broad concept of psychotropics as the range of pleasure-giving activities of the community for which some measure of unnatural drive (or dependence) exists. Examination shows that the rating order of the individual activities must represent the bias of the author. While the extremes can be labelled 'Deviant' and 'Normal' with ease, the limit of social acceptability depends upon a value judgement influenced by political, social and individual factors. Reproduced from Marks, J., *The Benzodiazepines*, 1978, Lancaster: MTP Press

As editors we expect to be criticized as biased in the selection of the topics and this criticism we readily accept. As we have explained above, we believe that subjective value judgements are involved in the definition of the social and medical problems of dependence. Living in another place or at another time our selection would surely have been quite different.

We have attempted to demonstrate the international nature of the problem by inviting contributions from experts from several different countries. The finding that not all experts contributing to this volume see eye to eye on all issues and problems touched upon only serves to underline the fact that so much in this field still awaits further elucidation, and that much more observation, research and interdisciplinary and international cooperation are required.

We believe, however, that there is a place for authoritative review and critical analysis of certain aspects of the problem written by observers with first-hand active and practical experience in their particular fields. This we have attempted to provide. Whether we have succeeded others must decide.

Max Glatt
John Marks

REFERENCES

Eddy, N. B. (1965). *Bull. WHO*, **32**, 721

Glatt, M. M. (1974). *A Guide to Addiction and its Treatment. Drugs, Society and Man.* (Lancaster: MTP Press)

Glatt, M. M. (1978). *Drug Dependence, Current Problems and Issues.* (Lancaster: MTP Press)

Marks, J. (1978). *The Benzodiazepines. Use, Overuse, Misuse, Abuse.* (Lancaster: MTP Press)

Smith, A. J. (1980). *Trends Pharmacology Sci.*, **August**

Stepney, R. (1980). *World Med.*, **September 23**

WHO (1957). Expert Committee on Addiction-producing Drugs. *7th Report. Tech. Rep. Ser.*, **116**

WHO (1969). Expert Committee on Drug Dependence. *16th Report. Tech. Rep. Ser.*, **407**

1

Pleasure-seeking and the aetiology of drug dependence

Wolfram Keup

Experiencing pleasure is one of the fundamental abilities for which living beings have the psychological capability. Being one of the strongest motivators of human behaviour, pleasure has been used by nature as a 'tool' to motivate living creatures throughout the developmental chain of animal life up to the highest primate, man. Without pleasure-seeking behaviour, higher life might long since have ended. Nature has been able – generation after generation – to entice animals and man to overcome lethargy, indifference and egocentricity, even to do laborious and painful work, to tackle dangerous and risky tasks in fulfilling superindividual functions such as the continuation of the species, rearing the young, seeking improvements in doing so – with pleasure as an expected reward. We are just beginning to learn about the biological mechanisms behind such behaviour, for example, from experiments in which animals are allowed to selfstimulate certain pleasure-generating areas of the brain, neglecting food, water and sex, continuing until there is complete exhaustion and sometimes even death (Olds, 1962). We know even less about the derangement of such biological mechanisms in addiction and similar pathological conditions.

Man – as well as some higher animals – has been capable of finding loopholes, obtaining pleasures without delivering natural superindividual tasks, then constructing concepts by which such behaviour appears not only justified but might even be cultivated, rationalizing his behaviour rather than adopting one which conforms with philosophical theory. Pleasure is felt by man to be such an important and basic part of his normal behaviour that the lack of the normal drive for pleasure fulfilment, or to be able to enjoy pleasures, is considered to be grossly abnormal. Thus, Rado (1957) considers the 'pleasure deficit' as one of the fundamental symptoms of schizophrenia.

Pleasure, though, has a wide range of phenotypes: the hearty eater, the voyeur, the body-building athlete, the scientist who sees his working hypothesis fulfilled, the power-wielding manager, the charitable moralist as well as the political fanatic starving himself to death – all have their own, very private kinds of pleasure fulfilment. In fact, almost any behaviour between total indulgence, total asceticism and total destruction or self-destruction can, by psychological processes, be converted into a pleasure.

Man indulging in 'unmerited' pleasures soon becomes conscience-stricken. The duration and the degree of pleasure it takes to reach this point vary widely, yet it seems that the lack of ensuing comfort not only represents the dys-ease with the moral issues of society and its value systems but an inborn braking mechanism against overindulgence and the neglect of other vital functions. Moral issues, though, play a considerable, even a decisive role, and the role of pleasure in life has surely been debated from time immemorial.

The Greek philosophers gave an example, variations of which re-emerged later throughout our cultural history.

Democritus (about 460–360 BC) saw 'euthymia', the supreme happiness, in a quiet and serene equilibrium of the soul, free from turmoil of passions, and based this on a steady flow of 'soul atoms', in the frame of a materialistic atomism. Socrates (about 469–399 BC), the venerated teacher and wise man representing and living a reason-ruled life in clear consciousness over the senses and affects, in full knowledge about 'eudaemonia', the true happiness from which all virtue originates, struck a balance between pleasure and control. Yet, while the master had accepted the cup of hemlock in dignity, his disciples battled in controversies over this issue. While Antisthenes (born about 430 BC) saw in the freedom, the independence from lust and pain, the rather puritan supremacy of the personality over these extremes, the highest goal of life, Aristippus (about 435–360 BC) postulated that joyfulness and pleasure (hedone) are the prime goals of human striving. Happy is a life only if it is rich in both physical and mental pleasures. 'Hedonism' bluntly postulated that good is what creates pleasures, although this was later mitigated by Epicurus (341–270 BC). These more extreme positions were somewhat bridged by a third disciple of Socrates, the more balanced Plato (427–348 BC): man cannot live by pleasure only; at the same time he strives for reason and insight, since otherwise he would live a dull and reduced life without remembrance and self-consciousness. These issues have, of course, been debated ever since with little chance of being solved entirely, since the answers cannot be fully binding for each independent individual in his own particular society. Thus, in almost every culture both liberal and puritanical attitudes exist side by side, with changing dominance.

Under the influence of these deep-rooted attitudes, pleasure-seeking and pleasure-withholding lie in precarious balance, and determined by many sociocultural factors, some of which are discussed below. Such influences, though, are changing with time, for example, religious beliefs, the cultural development, tolerance exercised towards the young, educational levels, cultural attitudes towards personal freedom and self-determination, etc. From such attitudes have resulted laws and rules regulating certain behaviours as allowable and 'normal', while outlawing and punishing other types of behaviour. Thus, opiates used for pleasure purposes are outlawed in our society, whereas alcohol is not, despite the latter being comparably harmful to individuals and to society. Sexual behaviour is outlawed only outside a certain framework which nevertheless shows a wide range of transcultural tolerances. Pleasures obtained from cruelty against animals are outlawed by all civilized populations, excluding matadors and fox hunters. There are strange lacunae in the way man justifies his behaviour which in themselves would be worth a study.

Pleasure has its price. Not only must it be earned by labour, endurance, suffering and renunciation at times, but it may encompass struggles to obtain it against competitors, the rules, the law, with the corresponding risks and consequences. It may be inseparable from deleterious effects upon physical and mental health – and its enjoyment may be followed by the displeasure of missing it, a dysphoria not at all restricted to substance abuse in general nor to substances to which physical tolerance develops. The longing for a beloved person is basically the same phenomenon as the craving for an addictive substance. But part of the displeasure quite often stems from the feeling of uneasiness with one's own conscience when delinquency is involved in obtaining pleasures, or the avoidance of dysphoria. This is even more pronounced when obsessive–compulsive tendencies are involved, as in dependence (consider the man who sends his girlfriend out to prostitute herself to obtain the money to support his habit!). Those suffering from substance abuse are not simply 'addicts', but men and women with the same personalities and vulnerabilities as the rest of us.

THE HISTORY OF SUBSTANCE ABUSE

It must be assumed that early man was already able to identify those plants yielding psychotropically active principles. A man, lost in the woods without weapons, would try roots and berries, chew leaves and tender young sprouts, thus experiencing their chemical effects. Or he would light a fire and inhale some of the smoke of an accidentally burned psychotropic plant, and hence experience its action (for example, cannabis as used by the Scythians). Thus, he would detect not only the nutritional value of roots and tubers but also the stimulating, sedating, appetite-reducing, psychotropic effects and toxicity of plant material. Hallucinations thus experienced are easily interpreted as voices of the gods; and the way to ritual use is paved. Even hallucinations and illusions due to hypoxia on mountain peaks have been used this way (among the Andean Indians). Almost without exception the ritual use of psychotropic substances precludes their abuse (alcohol in orthodox Jewish communities, mescaline in the 'Native American Church of North America', coca-leaf use in the early Inca culture, *Ilex vomitaria* used by North American Indians, and many others). The weakening of religious beliefs in the intellectualization of feelings and emotions tends to break down these forces. The age-old opposition of the young to the regimenting traditions of the elders, often simply used as a show of force by the young, favours this development (generation gap).

Increasing technical knowledge as well as de-ritualization has strongly influenced the spread of addictive substances. Two examples may be mentioned: the development of alcohol distillation which allowed inebriation with very small amounts of fluid. Distillation was described first in an arabic manuscript by Jäbir ibn Hayÿan (712–813 AD), but was forgotten again under the suppressive influences of Islam, to be rediscovered by the Franciscan monk Lully (about 1235–1315 AD) in southern France. Here, in favourable surroundings, it was refined and thus spread easily. A second example is the rapid spread of opiate dependence when the hypodermic needle, invented by Alexander Wood in 1853, was used for the subcutaneous and then intravenous injection of opiates, thus introducing what today is called the 'flash'. The use of cocaine yields the third example: whereas addiction in chronic coca-leaf chewers among the natives of South America leads only infrequently to severe dependence (cocaism), the extracted cocaine is one of our strongest dependence-producing substances (cocainism) (Austin, 1978; Nieschulz, 1969).

Only recently have we learned of yet another important step favouring misuse and dependence. In the course of development of his chemical knowledge in what was called the 'plastic age', man has become the creator of many new substances which are either (a) more addictive than their natural counterparts, (b) have new qualities, and/or (c) represent the addictive qualities in a pure way. As examples we may name highly potent yet equally addictive morphine derivatives and the many artificial hallucinogens like LSD-25, DMT (dimethyltryptamine), DET (diethyltryptamine), DOB (dimethoxybromoamphetamine), etc. Some like phencyclidine (PCP, Angel's Dust) display quite novel qualities dangerously close to the fundamental desires of man. It is obvious that currently the development of new agents occurs faster than the adaptational process by which man learns to deal safely with his creations. To achieve adaptation, it is not sufficient for the problem to be recognized by just a few, but it must be seen by a vast majority of the people so that self-restriction and voluntary controls by learning are popularized. Should man not learn to deal with present and future mind-influencing and mind-altering chemicals in time, he might soon find himself at the edge of an abyss. Manipulation of the emotions, of will-power, opinions and reduction of resistance against wrongs may lead to Chronos devouring his children, 'big brother' being the natural consequence.

AETIOLOGY OF DRUG ABUSE

It is not the purpose to discuss here how to deal with future threats, as briefly touched upon above. Instead, it is valid to return to the present and look at the many different factors and complex processes leading, often jointly, to substance abuse and particularly to drug abuse, dependence and its consequences.

Table 1.1 *Selective reasons for starting drug abuse (college students, New York City)*

Subjective reasons for starting drug abuse	*College students (New York, 1969)* n			%	
Sociological reasons					
Status-seeking	1				
Friends did it	64				
Influenced by relatives	1		68		18.7
Influenced by news media	1				
It's a drug-oriented society	1				
Psychological reasons					
For enjoyment	20	45		12.4	
For 'kicks'	25				
Out of curiosity		174		47.8	
As a challenge	3				
For new experience	8	36	275	9.9	75.6
As an experiment	25				
To escape, to forget	8				
For better insight	4	20		5.5	
Sick of drinking	3				
Out of boredom	5				
Medical reasons					
For weight loss	6				
To stay awake	2				
Against insomnia	1				
Against headaches	3		17		4.7
Against asthma	1				
Against depression	2				
Hospital-induced	2				
Other reasons					
War (Vietnam)	2		4		1.0
Coincidental circumstances	2				
All answers ($n = 605$)			364		100.0

SUBJECTIVE REASONS FOR BEGINNING DRUG ABUSE

People who abuse drugs have rather vague ideas about their own reasons for embarking on drug abuse. In 1972, we asked college students in New York City this question, among many others, and the 605 answers received while questioning 605 students are tabulated in Table 1.1. Among the reasons given are curiosity, inducement by friends, pleasure of experimenting, experience of 'kicks', and simply enjoyment, which rank highest. Other psychological reasons are rarely cited and those questioned seemed strikingly unaware of the psychological background upon which substance abuse developed.

When established drug users are seen at the initial interview for drug treatment, a great number of problems do surface, provided the interview is guided properly. All the misery of the life as an addict pours out, with its diminishing pleasure of developing tolerance and mounting problems of coping with side-effects, with the dysphoria of withdrawal, the many human problems involved in feeling forced to steal, to cheat and to prostitute, the crumbling of needed family ties, the deep distrust towards men in general and 'the man' in particular. Yet, very few correlations are made in these conversations, between these attitudes and the addict's personality or between his personality and the development of substance abuse and dependence. To make addicts aware of problems and to prepare the ground for therapeutic reasoning, we have used two simplified schematic drawings (Figures 1.1 and 1.2), which we discuss with the patient until he fully understands them, then ask him to localize his own problems in these drawings (Keup and Taegener-Torge, 1975).

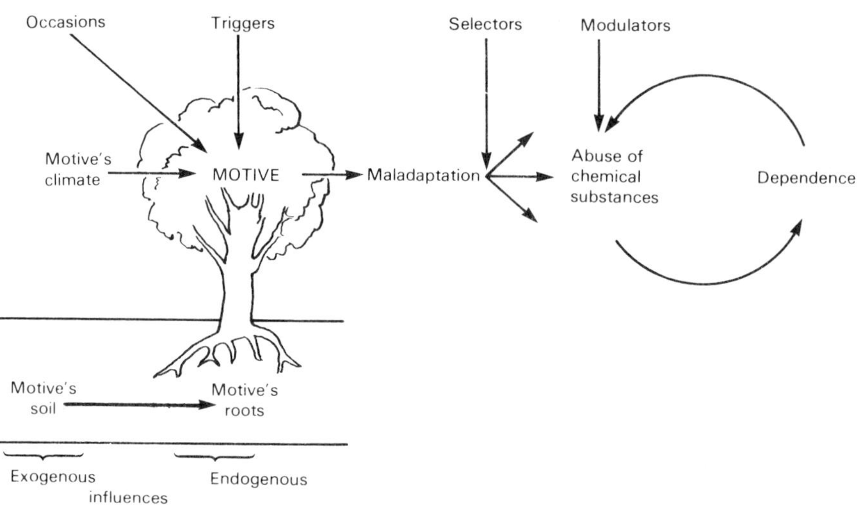

Figure 1.1 The 'motive tree' of drug abuse as a kind of maladaptation to life in family and community

The drug-dependent patient is usually fully aware of the fact that his substance abuse represents a maladaptation to the problems of life, but is unable to trace this back to its origins. We therefore tell him that there must have been a motive for him to act in this unusual way and that this motive might be compared to the crown of a tree, which has grown over many years; in other words, the motive has developed in his psyche as the result of a complex and branched process. The motive grew out of motivational roots which were able to grow the crown of the tree, because they were nourished by a motivational 'soil', furnished by the environment during the developmental years, mostly in childhood but sometimes later. To support the trunk and the crown of the tree, the motive could only develop in a motivational climate produced by the environment, such as school, neighbourhood, work, etc. Yet a mature motive for maladaptation becomes effective only when internal or external inductors trigger its action. In a series of investigations, we have seen that whereas objectively the most prominent factor lies in what is called the motivational soil, the family, and other environmental factors during the early years, the patients themselves tend to incriminate what is here called the motivational climate. They must also be made aware of the probability that the motive for maladaptation was non-specific and might have led to another type of deviant behaviour such as juvenile delinquency, sexual promiscuity, playing the role of a 'rocker' or a tramp, etc., and that the choice between these possibilities depends on many 'selectors' among which chance plays a major role. Once drug use has been selected, dependence does not inevitably follow, but instead a great many modulators, psychological as well as environmental, play a role in the development of what is discussed below as the 'drug career'. These later motivating forces are at times even more decisive – and therefore more important for therapy – than earlier ones. As mentioned above, the patient is often inclined to shift the blame from his own 'motivational tree' to environmental factors, a point at which we expose him to the complex involvement of his personality with the sociocultural environment (see Figure 1.3).

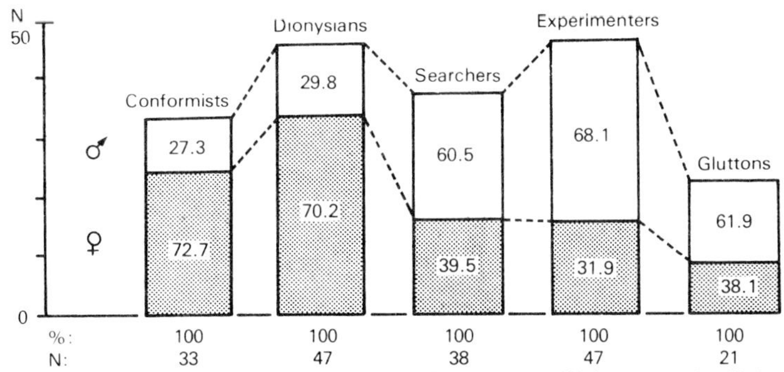

Figure 1.2 Relative frequency of motivational types for drug abuse among 186 college students with drug abuse (New York City)

Table 1.2 *Types of young drug-users according to their motive for drug abuse*

	Conformists	*Dionysians*	*Searchers*	*Experimenters*	*Gluttons*
Main motivation	To do what the group does, to share	Pleasure-oriented and social contact	Self-therapy attempt with some insight into sickness	Curiosity and intellectual reasoning	Pleasure-oriented, often emotional instability
Intelligence	Normal range, seldom better than average	Mostly medium intelligence, but of wide range	Mediocre, often limited	Often better than average	Often less than average
Social behaviour	Group-dependent (family-substitution), social contact	Good contact, also with permanence	Contact difficulties, 'lone wolf' – autism, often asocial	Social-minded, often assumes leading role, often without permanent partners	Good contact, but often without permanence, antisocial tendencies
Social class	All classes	Lower classes somewhat prevalent	Mostly from middle and lower classes	Often from middle and upper classes	All classes, lower classes somewhat prevalent
Psychological characteristics	Dependent, immature, leaning on others, in need of guidance, obstinate, lack of self-control	Light-hearted, carefree, pleasure-oriented, irrational, unbalanced, practical, extrovert, emotionally immature	Introvert, insecure, lacking ideas, dull, anxious, depression-prone	Active, without restraint, commanding, thorough, persevering, blustering, wilful, choleric	Aggressive, without discrimination, often lacking judgment, pleasure-oriented, often 'lone wolf', despotic, at times unsteady
Tendency towards progression and true dependence	Group-dependent, shies away from hard use, rarely true dependence	Slips easily into a full drug career, dependence is frequent	Changing slowly and systematically from one drug to the other. Danger of drug dependence relatively high	Tries systematically new drugs, applications, combinations. Relatively little danger of drug dependence	Distinct and frequent change, combinations. *Danger of overdose and high danger of drug dependence*
Psychiatric diagnosis	Corresponding to incidence in population. Little psychopathology	Endogenous psychoses and psychopathies not frequent. Moodiness. Juvenile reactions	Endogenous psychoses and prepsychotic states are frequent	Psychoses relatively rare. Protest reactions. Adaptation difficulties are frequent	Endogenous psychoses more frequent than with dionysians. Psychopathy prevails. Toxic psychoses not rare
Therapy	Detachment from the drug-scene, new interests. Readjustment of environment	Psychotherapy, group therapy. Possibly antidepressants	Antipsychotic, also psychopharmacological substitute for self-cure attempts through pointed psychiatric therapy	Intellectual promotion, remotivation towards better goals; good as teacher in AA-like programmes	Conscious adaptation to psychopathic symptoms sometimes feasible
Prognosis	Often good, also spontaneous recovery	Relatively good in most cases, Unfavourable in the case of 'pure' types. Often protracted recovery	Depending on basal psychopathology, but often relatively favourable as to abuse	Very wide range. Often better in case of good intelligence	Often unfavourable. 'Maturing-out' may be achieved

MOTIVATION FOR DRUG ABUSE

First, however, we ought to look at certain typical situations of motivation for drug abuse that are easily detectable in the histories of many drug users. These must not be misunderstood as representing personality types. Although much research has been carried out on distinct personality traits which predispose to chemical dependence, results have remained inconclusive (Keup, 1978). These motivational types show typical patterns of behaviour when originally in contact with drugs without having actually used them.

Table 1.2 reproduces the main characteristics of these types (Keup, 1972a and b). People falling into these typical patterns start drug abuse for quite different reasons. The 'searchers' are similar to 'problem drinkers' and have personal problems, anxieties, difficulties in concentration, lack of persistence. They are often shy and suffer from lack of contact, etc. In their early experiences with chemical substances they found relief from their symptoms; consequently they began a systematic search for the one particular compound that would best help them to overcome their problems. 'Dionysians', however, are driven by pleasure-seeking and the social contact derived from it. This makes them select drugs that are enjoyed within a group rather than a solitary situation, easing social contact. 'Experimenters' are driven by curiosity and the pleasure of encountering new experiences. They soon become very knowledgeable in the drug field and are often asked for advice by others. As a reward and to increase their pleasure they are often leaders of drug groups and so are rarely able to escape true dependence on strongly addictive substances such as opiates. 'Gluttons' have a rather unfavourable prognosis, since drug-taking in their case is the symptom of a more general instability and seducibility; they are fearless and reckless in the use of drugs and thus prone to overdose and intoxication. 'Conformists' are influenced by a peer group to take up drug abuse; often by a boy or girl friend; drug abuse in this group is a secondary motive, primary ones being seeking to be 'in' with the group, helping a friend, or simply being seduced to drug-taking under moral pressure. Their prognosis for treatment is better than that of all other groups, except for some of the 'searchers'. In this group, as in the 'dionysians', females prevail, but the opposite holds true in the three other groups. Figure 1.2 depicts the quantitative differences of the motivational types as investigated in a group of college students in 1969 (Keup, 1971; 1972b).

Not in all cases of drug abuse can a distinct type of motivation be detected. In our sample, 8.8% remained unassigned. In some of them, mixed motivation of two or more types was found.

THE TEXTURE OF SOCIOCULTURAL CONDITIONS

Before we return to the aetiological factors concerning personality, we should look at the involvement of people with their sociocultural

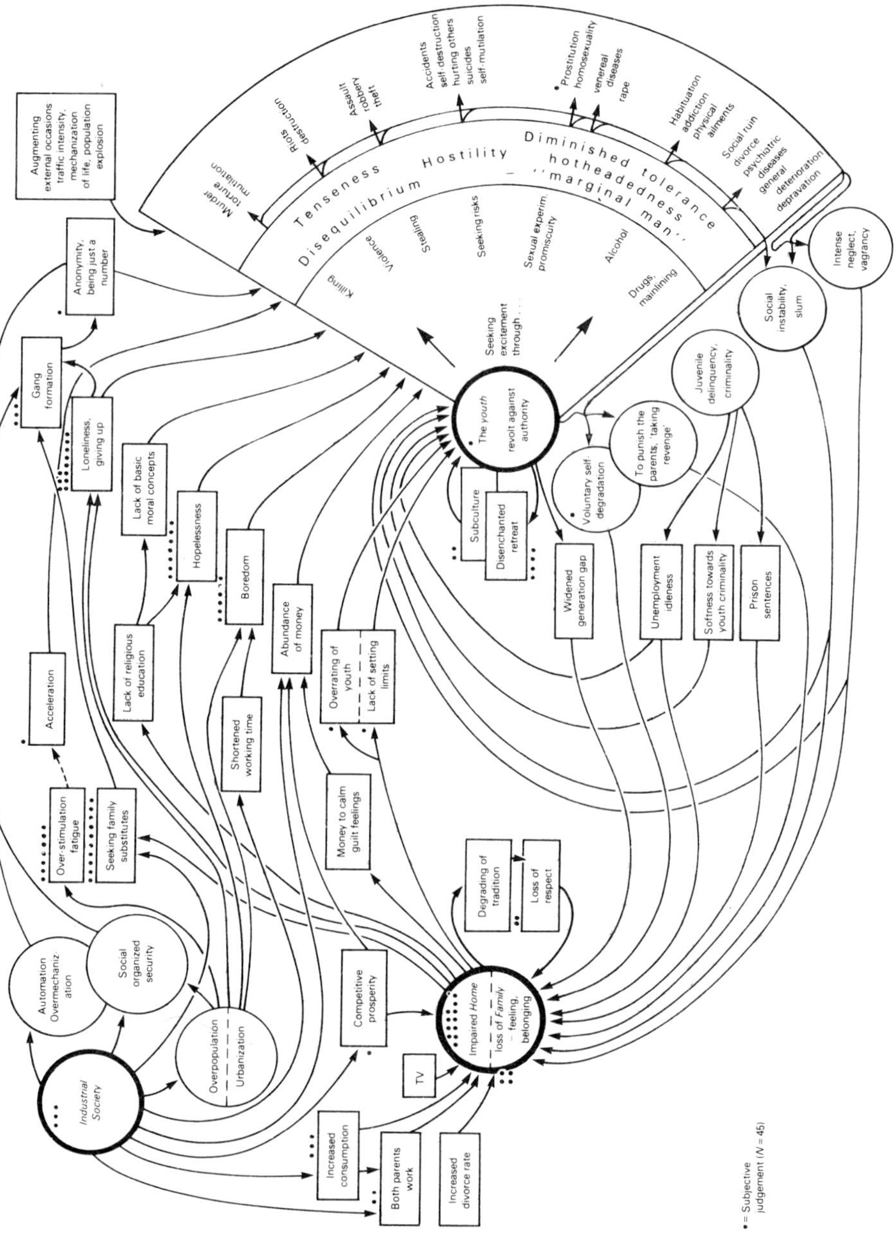

Figure 1.3 Sociocultural factors in the aetiology of maladaptation (with drug abuse) – the vicious circle of causative factors involving the family, the youth and 'industrial society'

environment. Figure 1.3 shows the schematic drawing used when the drug-addicted patient first comes for treatment (see above).

The drawing shows the many and complex relationships, causative or supplementary in the aetiology of drug abuse, often in the form of the vicious circle depicted (Keup, 1973). The cardinal points of the fine balance, which shifts towards disequilibrium before and during drug dependence, are: (1) the imbalanced, impaired home; (2) the young person himself or herself who has not found his or her natural place in either the family or the community; and (3) our present state of cultural development, complex in itself and here characterized by the rather simplified label of the 'industrial society'.

A family which fails to give security, shelter, and a climate of love and positive values to the children exposes them to many imbalanced influences both external and internal. Our life in 'industrial society' tends to overload people with information and unselected stimuli, and, although contacts tend to be pseudo-personal, they also tend to degrade the individual to a statistical entity. In our western world, the 'mature citizen' is supposed to know how to socialize, how to spend his leisure time, and how to develop his own inborn abilities without infringing on the rights of others. Young people, however, have to learn this, and they do so by exploring their capabilities on a trial-and-error basis. It is 'exploratory behaviour' which makes them test their abilities and strengths, following this path until they meet with resistance. This is a natural attitude we have in common with most living beings and risk-taking (Carney, 1971) during such endeavours is included. The liberality and an uncritical attitude towards what today is called freedom often sets a limit on these ventures too late, so repression and correction are used instead of early limitation. This has consequences which, in themselves, tend to widen the gap between the young and their families. The vicious circle closes. Under such complex conditions it becomes obvious that none of the classical models of drug addiction alone (Siegler and Osmond, 1968), such as medical, sociopsychological or moral, can explain the aetiology of drug dependence or even deviant behaviour in general. Under certain conditions they can in some individuals all be valid and are usually combined. To view this problem as originating from a 'super-pleasure' (Rado, 1957) alone, in analogy to the above-mentioned electrical self-stimulation experiments, seems barely justified (Blachly, 1970), nor does the theory that 'drugs are people substitutes' ('DAPS', see Blachly, 1970), although this might also play a role.

We must accept that there is no single cause for drug addiction, although typical kinds of conditions do exist at its onset. It also becomes evident that no single measure can ever be effective in preventing drug abuse, although we recognize two target areas: the family and its role in society as well as its inner climate; and the general attitude towards the use of chemical substances for comfort or the tolerance of discomfort.

We have, in standardized interviews, showed Figure 1.3 to drug-dependent patients and asked them to locate their troubles in this interrelated drawing (Keup and Taegener-Torge, 1975). The results are shown in Figure 1.3 as black dots. It is interesting that the family situation, either alone or in conjunction with influences from industrial society, is considered to be the most causative factor in starting a drug career.

ADAPTATIONAL CRISES

During his early development, man undergoes a number of changes which occur in a more or less regular pattern. It is interesting to note that maladaptation, followed by deviant behaviours, most frequently occurs at overlap points where there has to be adaptation to a new situation corresponding to a new level of maturity (Keup, 1973).

Early infancy, which is extrauterine in man only for the sake of brain development, is governed by the child's attempt to adapt totally to the mother and her physical as well as psychological feeding functions. At the end of the first year in which a strong 'psychological umbilical cord' still connects mother and child, the need for independence dawns; the first conflict is that between identification with the loved mother and her needs, and, on the other hand, the need to develop individuality.

In the early school years, tension mounts and self-restriction as well as adaptation to the needs of the family and the new school peer group are felt to be essential for a balanced existence. In middle childhood, a group of friends of the same age has been selected and firm relationships are established. Thus the first typical situation of overlapping interests is established, and conflict is imminent, since both this self-selected peer-group and the parental home are experienced as a positive basis for life, yet with conflicting demands. A time of controversial quickly changing decisions, ambivalence and depression results. This crisis is finally overcome by learning to cope with the demands of the group without any essential impairment of parental relationships; compromise is learned in the process. Yet, during this period, the child is very vulnerable to contact with enticing influences which promise quick solutions.

Two similar transitional periods exist at the beginning and the end of adolescence: the first is characterized by increasing lability and insecurity due to puberty with its many questions concerning the personality and its role in this world, at times culminating in 'identity crises'. The second transition is characterized by an overwhelming number of different roles as an adult in the 'establishment', induced by the feeling of belonging to the adult world. Adaptational difficulties in these overlapping situations are not at all rare. They have been estimated (Kysar, 1969) to exist in about 22% of college students. Some of these unbalanced young people behave as members of any minority would, as 'marginal men' (Levin). In this situation they easily identify with other minorities, be they racial, political or social, delinquent groups or drug-takers.

At the end of adolescence, an harmonious emancipation from th family has normally been reached. The adolescent has gained independ ence and a full capacity for psychological and sexual contacts, including the ability to develop lasting ties. Often, however, he or she, despite the ability to do so, does not immediately take on adult roles but lingers between preparedness and realization (phase of juvenility) (Keniston, 1970). This is accentuated by extended education, late marriage and certain phenomena of acceleration with early, and often incomplete, maturation.

Pleasure, leisure, freedom and satisfaction are goals, the meaning of which is experienced and recognized only slowly during the course of development. Although the bases for them are laid in early education, they can only be fully understood in adult life, yielding the ability to live by them when forced to decide along these lines. If the parents are immature themselves, catastrophe is inevitable. The inability of 'new religions' and sects, peer-groups and communes to function as family substitutes is obvious.

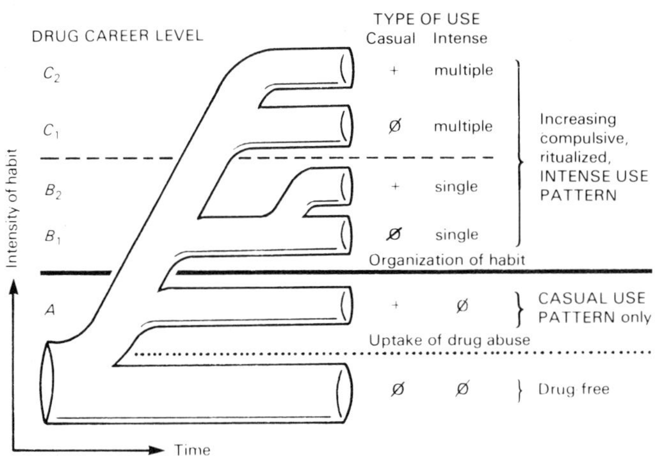

Figure 1.4 Steps and levels of a typical 'drug career'

THE DRUG CAREER

We have seen above that at the beginning of drug-taking, curiosity frequently becomes the initiating force compelling the person to overstep that first line of drug uptake – the initial use. Most of these curious people, however, soon abandon drug-taking after their curiosity has been satisfied. A true drug career starts, however, when the habit becomes regular and dependence has been established (Keup, 1971; 1972b). The line of 'organization of habit' (Figure 1.4) is the one borderline to be feared – at first the intense abuse pattern of just the drug alone, then with the added casual use of other substances. This develops still further with multiple intense use (polytoxicomania), and with other drugs added in casual use patterns, adds increasing difficulties to treatment. In the beginning, pleasure or the avoidance of displeasure plays a major role; later, it is euphoria with its drug-specific side-effects and the avoidance of dysphoria which is important. In fully developed opiate dependence, the avoidance of dysphoria and other withdrawal signs become the mainspring of continued abuse; pleasure is lost. For therapeutic purposes, it is important to know why the different steps have been taken by a particular patient (Keup, 1972b). If these motives are not recognized by the therapist and understood by the patient, there is the danger of transferring dependence to another object. Therapy, however is not our topic here.

COMMUNITY DEFENCES

So far, we have discussed in some detail three well-recognized major factors in the aetiology of drug abuse (see also Glatt, 1974); (1) the personality of the potential user, (2) his environment or social milieu, and (3) influences from the drug itself, such as time of uptake, dose–effect relationships, mode of application, ease of access, development of tolerance, the appearance of withdrawal symptoms, etc. This widely used triangular pattern is shown in Figure 1.5. Yet, to the customary triangular diagram (Kielholz and Ladewig, 1973) a fourth factor can be added which perhaps is often forgotten (Keup, 1981) – the defence capability of a cultural group or a country and its population against substance abuse and the ensuing dangers. If this reaction is strong enough, it can disrupt the necessary links between the three causative factors for a good many potential users, thus keeping the number of addicts small. This is not the place to describe this defence capability in detail, but it is composed of measures and controls issued by government; a sensible network of treatment facilities, and the necessary

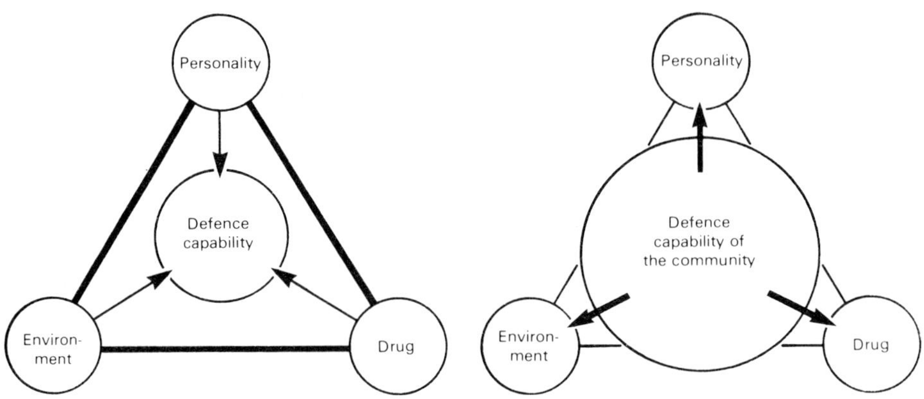

Figure 1.5 The role of awareness in and the defence capability of the community on the three basic groups of factors favouring the origin of drug abuse

institutions and systems to induce addicts to therapy. But probably mc important of all is the attitude of the population towards the abuse oı drugs, alcohol, medical drugs, nicotine as well as excesses in general. Transcultural factors, as well as political and attitudinal changes and concepts in a given population, play a major role. Here, of course, lie important possibilities for the prevention of drug-taking, but in it lie also the dangers of undue prudishness and Pharisaism as well as of a 'law-and-order society'.

TYPICAL PHASES OF A 'DRUG WAVE'

The defence capability is slow in developing when, in the course of a 'drug wave', a country is forced to deal with this problem. The response, however, follows a distinct pattern which is outlined in Table 1.3 (Keup, 1980).

The term 'drug wave' implies that the crest is followed by a decline. Signs are beginning to appear in some countries of the western world that this is in fact occurring, but we cannot be sure yet. The danger in this development lies in the temptation, appearing regularly during the management phase, to accept substance abuse as an irrevocable fact of every day life and to learn to live with it. Hence it is managed simply as is any other phenomenon of life, instead of uncovering the causes and fighting them. Only then can it be hoped that a sixth phase will follow: the 'phase of restoration' with drastic reduction of the problem. And only then is the term 'drug wave' justified.

CONCLUSIONS

Pleasure represents a natural and a vital quality of life. Pleasure-seeking behaviour thus has a firm basis and is fully justified. Nature uses this quality to reach certain goals, to entice man to do tasks that would otherwise charge him with duties and responsibilities requiring work and endurance. Biology even goes further. Under some circumstances, the threshold for obtaining pleasures is raised. It has to be earned, obtained against competition, at times by painful compromise, involving manipulation and secrecy – yet, the feeling of pleasure can be enhanced by the fact that it is hard to obtain. Frustration increases the drive to obtain it and pleasure seems biologically to be the reward for the strongest. Yet, man has been able to obtain many pleasures for free, though he overlooks the fact that for this ability too he pays a price. Permanent pleasure is no pleasure anymore; and to maintain the feeling of pleasure under such conditions, the pleasure-intensity must be raised or new qualities added to re-establish the figure –ground relationship. This, then, is not only a peculiarity of tolerance-producing drugs; it also holds true in others, such as in cocaine dependence and is not even necessarily restricted to drugs. If we do not recognize that we are tied to such principles by the simple fact that we are living beings, then we put man against nature. But it must be assumed

Table 1.3 *The phases of development of a typical 'drug wave' independent of local and national conditions*

Phases, characteristics	*Substances typical for each phase*
0–**Latency phase** Rise of abuse/dependence up to a problem threshold embedded in other social problems	no specific substances, local differences, opiates or stimulants, at times sleeping pills, analgesics
1–**Ideological phase** Shock-phase, poor reaction from government and other responsible authorities Ideological controversies, politically influenced Society is blamed; glorification of the 'user' Unrealistic tolerance Beginning of organized 'self-help' groups	cannabis (hashish, marijuana) LSD-25 and other hallucinogens, 'uppers' and 'downers' from the family medicine-chest
2–**Phase of overestimation** Overreaction on the part of government, laymen-organizations and the 'establishment' Methadone-maintenance programmes (substitution) discussed Beginning of official counteraction first professional therapy programmes, still not very effective	opiates – heroin 'Speed' (amphetamines and related agents); cocaine as secondary substance, sometimes 'therapy' – attempts with methadone, tilidine, etc.; these appear on the black market
3–**Therapy-phase** Drug-free programmes prevail Help offered at all costs! Professionals take over lead in counter-measures Ideological aspects fade Drugs no more 'in', less fashionable Polytoxicomania, involvement of women increase A change to alcohol becomes more frequent The 'drug-scene' goes underground, but dealing intensifies	heroin and numerous changing substitutes, also alcohol, hard-use patterns begin to take over from casual abuse
4–**'All-clear'-phase** Officials tend to consider the problem as solved Financial support stops; the experts have difficulties to overcome this problem Drug problem becomes an issue in political power struggles Preventive measures slowly become more effective The 'hard core' of addicts grows under a mask Criminality increases; more deaths Fierce competition on the black market, merging with prostitution (pimps) Decentralization and 'privatization' of the drug trade First, curiosity disappears, then the public interest	heroin is the leading drug; again hashish and LSD; solvent sniffing; other, more exotic substances; alcohol, abused like a drug; distinct 'drug careers' methadone (MMP) is again discussed
5–**Management-phase** Data collections furnish realistic picture: efficiency controls Success of programmes is judged more objectively Diversified therapy offers homes, after-care Cost/efficiency analyses Minimum requirements for therapeutic institutions	heroin and other opiates; cannabis preparations; cocaine, as primary substance; ephedrine and other stimulating drugs

Table 1.3 *(Continued)*

Polyvalent abuse now is the rule, including alcohol Polytoxicomania reaches an upper level Motivation for therapy becomes the central issue Jurisdiction adapts to these requirements Care for therapy-resistant addicts is being recognized as a necessary task Therapy-chains, or nets are being organized	also: psychoactive medical drugs, and drugs of all sorts alcoholism is an 'escape' from drugs

that man has not changed mentally in the past 60 000 years or so, and anybody who thinks man can change his emotion-ruled attitudes from one generation to the next simply by recognizing the way he ought to go, is denying the biological animal we, in many respects, still are. We will overcome this only thousands of years hence.

Pleasure, then, is only the exception and is felt only against the background of lack of pleasure, even displeasure, pain, depression, hard work, grinding routine and occasional dysphoria. Happiness is not a human right but an exceptional gift – it cannot be made a permanent state. Misery is not abolished by happiness, pleasure and euphoria but by doing something positive to combat it. Of course, this will mean work, sweat and endurance – but at the end, it may also mean **satisfaction**, a quality of life quite different from pleasure. Nowadays 'work is done for money only, never for the satisfaction of a job well done. Enjoying one's work is something we dare not mention for fear of castigation in a pleasure-bent social milieu' (Berger, 1972).

We hear much these days of self-fulfilment and self-realization without anybody telling us what the 'self' should be like. It needs to be re-established that a job well done, a responsibility borne successfully, a durable and useful piece of handicraft produced, a productive thought to the betterment of a situation put into action, living up to one's promise, being of use and of help to other people, generates satisfaction. Of course, the positive value of work is viewed by some as being outmoded, belonging to a bygone era. Yet whereas pleasure diminishes with repetition, satisfaction grows with it. Have you ever seen a satisfied drug-user? Talking to drug-dependent people, one is often horrified to see that they do not have any idea of the interconnection of human qualities – nobody has ever told them. No wonder that they are wide open and receptive to 'new religions' and sects which do not give them freedom of decision but pseudo-idealistic ideas packaged in dependence instead. Young people nowaday *are* receptive. They have strong religious desires, and even ascetic tendencies or at least a drive for a simple, more direct and basic life can be observed among them. But all this needs to be channelled to their own benefit, to the benefit of society at large and, finally, of us all. There are no simple solutions to the problem of drug abuse as there are none to the many questions of educating the young. The 'pleasure deficit' felt by young people in our society, feeling 'ill at ease with the world', prepares the way for the development and spreading of substitutes, promising instant gratification yet withholding it at the end. Only in the beginning is there pleasure involved in drug-taking. With opiates and other drugs there is in a very short time the seesaw mechanism between euphoria and withdrawal. With hallucinogens (Hicks, 1972; Katz, 1968), alcohol and medical drugs, similar conditions exist. In the end it is the avoidance of dysphoria, physically induced or not, which prolongs addiction. But it must be said that dysphoria itself is a necessary part of addiction, since permanent euphoria would neither be tolerable nor would it last; dulled as it is by time it would require new highlights or the background of its opposite both being part of the process of dependence.

Pleasure, of course, has an important role in life, as we have already pointed out. But some individuals, cultures, epochs, have difficulty in sensing the borderline between use of chemical substances and their misuse or abuse. This borderline is, indeed, hard to describe. It can probably best be sensed by comparing the following three pairs of chemical substances: (1) coffee versus cocaine, (2) alcohol versus barbiturates, and (3) cannabis versus heroin. Caffeine has a medical effect, particularly useful in older people, and, as a stimulant of the central nervous system, it eases communication and certain mental processes. Wherever it occurs in nature it has been found even by primitive peoples and used without abuse developing, although in history it has been pursued by prohibition. Overdose as well as chronic overuse are detrimental, and intoxication as well as rare dependence can be harmful. Cocaine, another stimulant, also has remedial faculties, but its toxicity and addiction potential far outweigh any justifiable psychological effect.

Alcohol and barbiturates belong to the same group as far as addiction is concerned, the WHO barbiturate/alcohol-type. Both are strongly toxic. Alcohol causes more tissue toxicity, whereas barbiturates have a rather small margin of safety as to vital brain centres. If we were faced with the question whether or not to introduce alcohol as a medical drug today, the substance certainly would be turned down because of its toxicity. But it is 'socially accepted' and, in limited use, is thought by many to have a social function though this is denied by others. Pharmacologically though, its safety margin is certainly too narrow, and many a user is unable to keep within this margin, to control a safe uptake. Barbiturates, similar to morphine, have no defensible social function nor have they any psychological benefit for the user. In addition, their addiction potential is high while withdrawal can be life-threatening.

Cannabis, abused by millions of people in this world, might provide some 'pleasure', but the lifestyle that goes with it leads to a dead-end socially and mentally. For the western world, it is a good model for what we have said about the alternative between pleasure and satisfaction. Moreover, research has to date no final answer on the dangers involved in cannabis abuse, but lately data on deleterious effects have started to accumulate. Heroin has no properties that might improve the quality of life, the ability to be of help to others, or to improve those faculties of life which enable man to cope with the problems of this world, of his upkeep and of his duties towards others, his children, his grandparents, and society at large.

Marks (1978) has tried to place pleasure-yielding principles of our culture in a system of coordinates of social acceptability and dependence. Although this establishes a valuable rough hierarchy, the relative place in it very much depends on *how* a given 'pleasure' is obtained. Thus, certain sexual behaviour can acquire the quality of a dependence as well as certain obsessive–compulsive attitudes too. On the other hand, even 'narcotics' are used in many patterns and for many different purposes. Alcohol may be used in a wide range of ways, from 'normal' social drinking to overwhelming and very harmful dependence with deviant behaviour – its location in a hierarchy depending on 'set and setting' of its use and the many other influences briefly described in this paper. Additional dimensions and coordinates would then be needed for a complete 'location' of pleasures.

Judging these differences, of course, can only be subjective. But we do have to be subjective, independent and opinionated. We do need personalities. We do need people willing and able to guide the young into a humane and productive direction, if man is to prevail. We do need to re-establish a rather simple, perhaps rural, attitude towards what life is all about, what relative place pleasure has, and what the terms duty and self-fulfilment really represent, meanwhile, of course, not punishing pleasure, but recognizing its true value in life and its limitations.

Drug abuse might be treated by weaning a person from the substance abused, but this is no treatment for the underlying causes that have led him or her to substance abuse. Only if these causes and conditions are remedied, is there a chance that relapse, or transition to another similar pathological behaviour, can be avoided. For this, the explanation of the difference between pleasure and satisfaction, the mental understanding of this difference and the acceptance of it with the heart are certainly the most essential steps to be taken.

REFERENCES

Austin, G. A. (1978). Perspectives on the history of psychoactive substance use. *NIDA Research Issues*, **24**, (Washington DC: US DHEW)

Berger, H. (1972). Compulsory education – a cause of drug addiction. In Keup, W. (ed.) *Drug Abuse, Current Concepts and Research*. pp. 171–9 (Springfield: Charles C. Thomas)

Blachly, P. H. (1970). Seduction. *A Conceptual Model in the Drug Dependencies and Other Contagious Ills*. (Springfield: Charles C. Thomas)

Carney, R. E. (1971). *Risk-taking Behaviour*. (Springfield: Charles C. Thomas)

Glatt, M. M. (1974). *A Guide to Addiction and its Treatment*. (Lancaster: MTP Press)

Hicks, R. E. (1972). Pleasurable and unpleasurable feeling states in hallucinogenic drug experience. In Keup, W. (ed.) *Drug Abuse, Current Concepts and Research*, pp. 135–45. (Springfield: Charles C. Thomas)

Katz, M., Waskow, I. and Olsson, J. (1968). Characterizing the psychological state produced by LSD. *J. Abnorm. Psychol.*, **73**, 1

Keniston, K. (1970). Postadolescence (youth) and historical change. In: Zubin, J. and Freedman, A. (ed.) *Psychopathology of Adolescence.* pp. 34–50 (New York: Grune and Stratton)

Keup, W. (1971). The typical 'drug career' and therapeutic approaches. *Proceedings of the 33rd Annual Meeting, Committee on Problems of Drug Dependence.* pp. 1049–63 (Toronto: National Research Council, National Academy of Science)

Keup, W. (1972a). Differences in therapy for drug users according to their motive for abuse. In Keup, W. (ed.): *Drug Abuse, Current Concepts and Research.* pp. 397–406. (Springfield: Charles C. Thomas)

Keup, W. (1972b). Die Psychopathologie jugendlicher Drogenabhängiger – Ansätze zur Therapie. In: DHS (ed): *Drogen- und Rauschmittel-Missbrauch. Schriftenreihe zum Problem der Suchtgefahren. Heft. 17*, pp. 71–86. (Hamm: Hoheneck-Verlag)

Keup, W. (1973). Krisen der individuellen Anpassung. In Schlemmer, J. (ed.). *Anpassung als Notwendigkeit.* pp. 94–105. (München: Piper Verlag)

Keup, W. (1973). *Nachreifung als Therapieziel bei jugendlichen Drogenabhängigen.* (Kassel: Nicol-Verlag)

Keup, W. (1978). Zur Typologie der Suchtentstehung. In Keup, W. (ed.). *Sucht als Symptom.* pp. 68–81. (Stuttgart: Thieme Verlag)

Keup, W. (1980). Die Entwicklungsgeschichte einer 'Drogenwelle' im Vergleich der Nationen. *Medica*, **1**, Sonderheft 32–33

Keup, W. (1981). *Abhängigkeitsentstehung und Drogen-Karriere.* (Bonn: Das Parlament), **31**, 33, p. 3

Keup, W. and Taegener-Torge, Ch. (1975). Ätiologie des Missbrauchs aus objektiver und subjektiver Sicht. In Keup, W. (ed.): *Missbrauch chemischer Substanzen – neuere Forschungsergebnisse.* pp. 51–8 (Hamm: DHS)

Kielholz, P. and Ladewig, D. (1973). *Die Abhängigkeit von Drogen.* p. 24. (München: dtv-Wiss. Reihe)

Kysar, J. E. *et al.* (1969). Range of psychological functioning in 'normal' late adolescents. *Arch. Gen. Psychiatry*, **21**, 515

Marks, J. (1978). *The Benzodiazepines. Use, Overuse, Misuse, Abuse.* p. 10. (Lancaster: MTP Press)

Nieschulz, O. (1969). Kokaismus und Kokainismus. *Münch. Med. Wochenschr.*, **111**, 2276

Olds, J. (1962). Hypothalamic substrates of reward. *Physiol. Rev.*, **42**, 555

Rado, S. (1957). Narcotic bondage: A general theory of the dependence on narcotic drugs. *Am. J. Psychiatry*, **114**, 165

Siegler, M. and Osmond, H. (1968). Models of drug addiction. *Int. J. Addict.*, **3**, 3

2
Legislation on drug control and drug abuse

John H. Langer

Efforts to control the use of psychoactive substances have been recorded since earliest times. In the classical Greek and Roman periods, mention is made of alcohol excesses, and in Asia Minor and Assyria even earlier use of cannabis is described. Opium, primarily as a medicine, was also known and used, and introduced into China and India in the 8th and 9th centuries. By 1250, alcohol was being distilled in Europe, and also used for medicinal purposes. The Incas of South America were using coca leaves in ritual ceremonies in the 14th century. By this time coffee, cultivated first in Ethiopia, had spread through the Middle East.

By the 16th century, world trade had carried drugs and psychoactive substances to most of the then-known world. The intermingling of cultures ruptured the traditional social and religious controls and a new era of experimentation and adventure ensued, part of which was the use of potent new and exotic substances: tea from China, tobacco, cocoa and coca from the Americas, coffee from the Middle East. The evolution from medicinal drugs to abuse of drugs for many of these natural substances can be traced, and the efforts to stamp out their subsequent abuse has been described in detail in numerous publications.

Common historical routes taken by present-day drugs of abuse are the medical and the ritual. A substance is first identified as a medication, then promoted as beneficial and not habituating, and finally found to be widely abused and in fact dependence-creating. In the ritual route, in largely homogeneous societies, the moral perspective of community leaders sets the tone for the society. Rules or religious taboos prohibiting, restricting or regulating the substance and its use were readily accepted, even if not always obeyed, until the intrinsic controls had broken down. Sometimes the same substance is involved in both routes, as for example opium, cocaine and cannabis. An objective study of this phenomenon in different societies would be useful for present and future control efforts.

By the 20th century, the world had seen the opium wars between China and England; suppression of tobacco, hashish, coffee, tea, and alcohol, as well as the opiates in many countries; the development of an increasing interest in medicines, and an accompanying effort to regulate or control them by religious reformers as well as governments and professional medical authorities.

The failure of many efforts to suppress addictive substances need not be chronicled here. The availability of alcohol, tobacco, coffee, cocoa and tea reveal the strength of man's desire to stimulate or sedate himself, even at the expense of his health. Yet some drugs *were* controlled. The opiates, cocaine, and cannabis were all effectively controlled in many places for considerable periods of time. The common factors in earlier successes in controlling these substances may be instructive for this discussion, if they can be identified. However, in modern times the manufacture and distribution of synthetic and semi-synthetic psychoactive substances have given rise to additional and entirely new issues of regulation and control for modern society.

Effective control of modern drug legislation presupposes the existence of high technology, an efficient long-distance transport system and a sophisticated economic and social milieu. Unfortunately, governmentally legislated control methods and techniques have not kept pace with technology and financial advances. There is easy movement of drugs in high demand–with high financial incentives for trading–across natural boundaries, national borders and then to the retail market. Instantaneous communication, easy transfer of money, and rapid world-wide transportation are the tools of the illicit trafficker in drugs. Drugs control legislation which does not take into account the uses of these tools is ineffective; unless the enforcement and regulatory agencies charged with control have sufficient manpower, finance and expertise to discover the methods of shipment and payment, follow them to their sources, identify the lawbreakers and successfully prosecute them, drug control legislation is useless. The present most common method, harassment by police of users and low-level dealers is a perpetuation of an outmoded system. It is still in use because the abuse of drugs, legal and illegal, has only recently exploded on the consciousness of societies and the large numbers of people involved reported in the mass media only in the past few years. Police methods and resources have not kept pace. There are exceptions. In countries or areas where the control agencies can in fact exert deterrent pressure on the user, drug use is low. This, of course, requires awareness of the public and actual punishment or other sanction sufficient to deter.

The present situation in drug legislation appears, in oversimplified terms, to be the following: there is in place a generally coherent system of international, national and local control based on conventions, national laws and local ordinances. These define objectives, describe what is to be controlled, define the roles of the respective executive agencies, and establish a framework for the administration of regulations and civil and criminal penalties. This system is more or less effective depending upon a complex set of factors which are described below.

The United States Department of State conducted a survey of drug controls in 1978 and 1979 which, although incomplete, indicates that there is in fact a worldwide system of control based on national legislation dealing with limitations and penalties in most countries for possession, distribution, cultivation, production, and financing dealings involving the controlled substances (Bureau of International Narcotics and Matters, 1979).

Controls on psychoactive substances have evolved through national and international regulation in many ways, formal and informal. It must be understood that in modern societies social and legal controls are so complex that they often conflict, especially where the substances have both accepted and proscribed uses, or where legal and social constraints are contested or ignored by some members of a society. The resultant conflict can force re-evaluation of the objectives of the laws controlling the substances, the methods of control, financial needs for control of the substance and those using it, and require programmes for re-education of the public.

Table 2.1 *Taxonomy of the types of control and related aspects. Source: Blum et al.* (1974)

1 EXPLICIT DRUG LAW OBJECTIVES

Revenue supply
- taxation
- licensing
- monopolies
- records

Consumer health and protection
- licensing requirements for production and sales
- drug purity
- advertising controls
- prescription requirements
- monopoly control
- proofs of drug efficacy
- proofs of drug safety
- warnings as to toxicity
- protection of special religious (drug) practices
- price controls
- labelling as to contents and dosage
- provision for low-cost distribution as part of public medical care delivery
- support for research and development

Prevention of abuse
- elimination of drug supply
  - prohibitions on possession and use
  - prohibitions on sales
  - prohibitions on associations or places of association
  - penalties to deter abuse
  - crop situation
  - precursors

Table 2.1 *(Continued)*

religious law (sanctions by or in support of)
restriction on drug supply
licensing of sellers
limitations on supply
(state) monopolies
record keeping
licensing of distributors (physicians, scientists, etc.)
licensing of research workers and establishments
prescriptions
religious law (sanctions by or in support of)
quotas
education
support for research
Rehabilitation
civil commitment
criminal commitment
compulsory reporting of addicted persons
education and advertising
obligation to undergo treatment
obligation to provide treatment
provision of social welfare or other support
Organization and administration
authorizing and defining the functions (structures of administrative bodies)
funding administrative organs
retail dealers of psychoactive substances (other than pharmacists)
researchers, dentists, veterinarians, etc.
taxation
limitations
limitation on time of sale
limitation on age of buyer
limitation on place of sale
limitation on amount of sale
advertising
prohibition
review and limitations
warnings
import/export laws
prohibition
licences
records
monopolies
taxation
limitations to certain ports
quotas
consumer controls
prohibition of use
registration of user
age limitations
time limitations
place of use limitations

- limitations of amount used
- activity limitations

research and development controls

- defining research activities, research workers, and establishments
- stipulating research substances and their uses
- stipulating research subjects and safeguarding procedures

2 FOCUS OF CONTROL

Raw materials

- agricultural controls
  - prohibition laws
  - licensing laws
  - government monopolies
  - taxation laws
  - crop substitution

Chemical precursors

- chemicals/materials used in manufacture

Manufacture

- prohibition of manufacture
- licensing
- monopolies
- labelling
- drug purity laws
- inventories
- taxation
- quotas

Distribution

- sales
  - prohibition
  - licensing
    - consumer
    - physicians
    - pharmacists
    - wholesale distributors
    - other suppliers of psychoactive substances
    - researchers
    - dentists, veterinarians, midwives, etc.
  - monopolies
  - record-keeping
    - physicians
    - pharmacists
    - wholesale distributors

3 TREATMENT LAWS

Compulsory reporting to government of addicted persons

- civil commitment
- criminal commitment
- treatment enabling legislation (establishing programme, facilities, and funding)
- legislation restricting treatment to particular physicians, clinics, or other especially licensed entities
- legislation defining eligibility for treatment
- legislation requiring mandatory tests to detect users.

Table 2.1 *(continued)*

4 PREVENTION: EDUCATION
Education in the schools
optional drug education
compulsory drug education

Drug education and professionals
Media
Warnings
Compulsory education of the citizenry

A comprehensive taxonomy of the types of control and related aspects is provided in Blum *et al.* (1974, p. 73) (see Table 2.1). It is testimony to the advances of technology in trade, transportation and communication that the countries of the world are generally agreed on which psychoactive substances need to be controlled. Illicit drug traffickers have never respected political boundaries, and international control requirements have increased as new technology has made them necessary.

The 1909 International Opium Commission which met in Shanghai examined the problem of narcotics trafficking, and was the first effort to involve a large number of countries. The first meeting resulted in nine resolutions which influenced the Hague Convention of 1912 and whose influence is still found in the 1971 Convention of Psychotropic Substances. Full descriptions of the development of international agreements are widely available and will not be repeated here. As controls became more widely accepted, the League of Nations and then the United Nations assumed responsibility for administration of the agreements. Present international narcotics and dangerous drugs controls encompass measures for control, information, action by the International Narcotics Control Board, and the promotion of prevention and rehabilitation.

Table 2.2 *Range of controls*

REQUIRE PARTIES TO CONTROL NARCOTICS AND DANGEROUS DRUGS
To prohibit, limit and/or control production-manufacture (legal)
total quantity produced
location of production
licensing of producers
regulation of amount each producer can produce
crop substitution
To control traffic (legal)
registration of wholesale traffic and distribution
sale only to government
To control utilization, consumption and stocks
statistics
certification
To enact and enforce criminal laws respecting narcotics and dangerous drugs
cultivation, production and manufacture (illegal)
trafficking (illegal)
possession and use (illegal)

REQUIRE PARTIES TO SUBMIT INFORMATION TO INTERNATIONAL BOARD
To submit yearly statistics (legal)
 production-manufacture
 traffic-internal, export, import
 utilization in manufacture of other drugs
 consumption
 stocks
To submit yearly estimates (legal)
 estimates of requirements
 estimates of amount to be produced or manufactured
To submit enforcement information
 laws and regulations
 seizures of illicit drugs
 arrests
To submit non-medical/scientific usage information
 estimates of traffic
 estimates of usage and addicts
To submit information on drug-abuse prevention and rehabilitation
 education-prevention programme
 rehabilitation programmes (medical, psychological, social, vocational)

EMPOWER BOARD TO TAKE ACTIONS
To request further information from parties
To request explanations from parties
To make public announcements
To suggest local inquiry
To make local inquiries with consent
To recommend embargo
To announce and impose embargo

PROMOTE PREVENTION AND REHABILITATION
 assistance to other nations
 education efforts through UN organs
 regional centres

An outline describing the range of controls is provided in a US government study of drug control by international treaty (Bureau of Narcotics and Dangerous Drugs, 1972; see Table 2.2). The present international system of narcotics control is the culmination of a series of control efforts, primarily through multilateral treaties. The bases for the present international control system are the 1961 Single Convention on Narcotic Drugs, and the 1971 Vienna Convention on Psychotropic Substances.

There are many technical aspects in the two major agreements. These give rise to limitations imposed by the agreements themselves, as well as exceptions taken by individual countries, as permitted by the agreements. The signatories bring their national laws into consistency and consonance with the international agreements.

CRITERIA FOR DRUG CONTROL LEGISLATION

To be effective laws must be acceptable to and accepted by those who are to be controlled by them. The laws must be promulgated effectively so that those affected understand the limitations placed on them and others, their rights and responsibilities, and the sanctions (penalties) for breaking the law. According to criminologists, for the law to be effective, those who come under it must believe that they will suffer penalties if they violate it, and they must know that the law is administered consistently, even if it appears harsh or unfair.

Beyond the criteria of reasonableness, consistency, fully promulgated, and effectively communicated, there are special characteristics required of laws which control drugs, drug dispensers and sellers, and drug users. These characteristics differ with the varying situations in countries, communities, and other political subdivisions. They also differ with the target – the part of the population the law is designed to control. The major factor in the control equation is control of the activities of those who in some way themselves have access and control of a drug – licit or illicit.

Where the drug is processed from organic material – plants or naturally formed matter – those who control the raw material are a natural focus of control. Thus, poppy-growers, coca-plant cultivators, and marijuana farmers are of special concern to those who administer and enforce the laws dealing with those substances. From the grower and harvester the substance moves to the processer, who makes the substance less bulky and more usable, and then to the distributor, who disperses the drug through the distribution network. Through this network it reaches the retail seller and then the user.

This process, though simple in description, involves many different activities. The manufacture of synthetic drugs differs in the initial stages of raw materials processing, but bulk and dosage unit manufacturing, wholesaling and retail distribution are similar. The user obtains the amount of drugs he needs or wants, limited by availability and the amount of money required. Figures 2.1 and 2.2 describe the movement of drugs from the source to the consumer. Figure 2.1 describes the movement of both controlled substances which are legally manufactured as well as synthetic or semisynthetic drugs in the illicit market. There is a marked similarity in the processes. However, the illicit market has no controls other than the legal restrictions and penalties incurred when those engaged in illegal activities are apprehended and convicted. Figure 2.2 shows illegal organic drug processing from the grower to the illicit market. There are no controls at any level, similar to the illicit market in synthetic substances, shown in Figure 2.1, but the figure does not show what occurs when drugs are diverted at various points in the processing from legal to illegal channels. In fact the channels described in Figure 2.2 show how legally produced but diverted drugs are handled – once they are in illicit channels both synthetic and organic licit and illicit drugs move to the drug abuser in

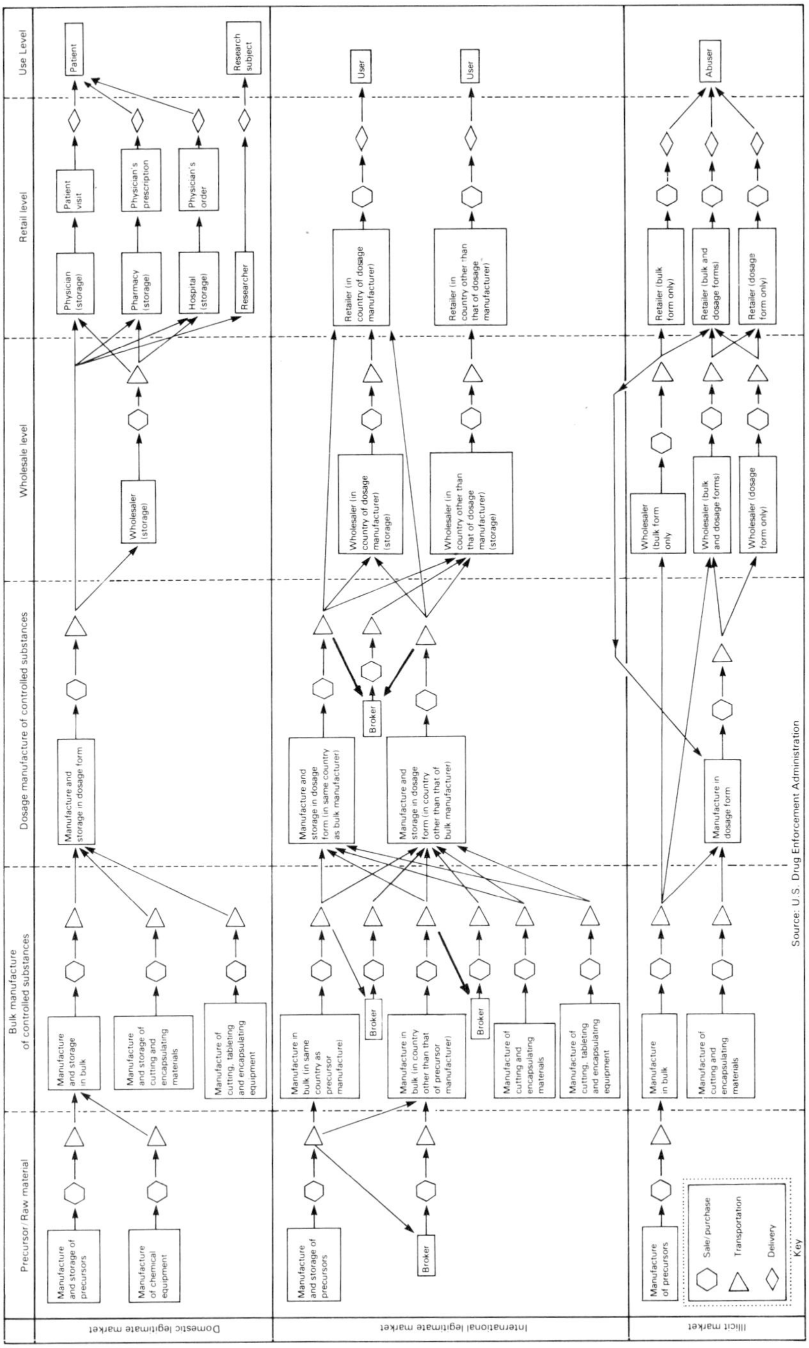

Figure 2.1 Legal and illicit drug movement from sources to users. Source: US Drug Enforcement Administration

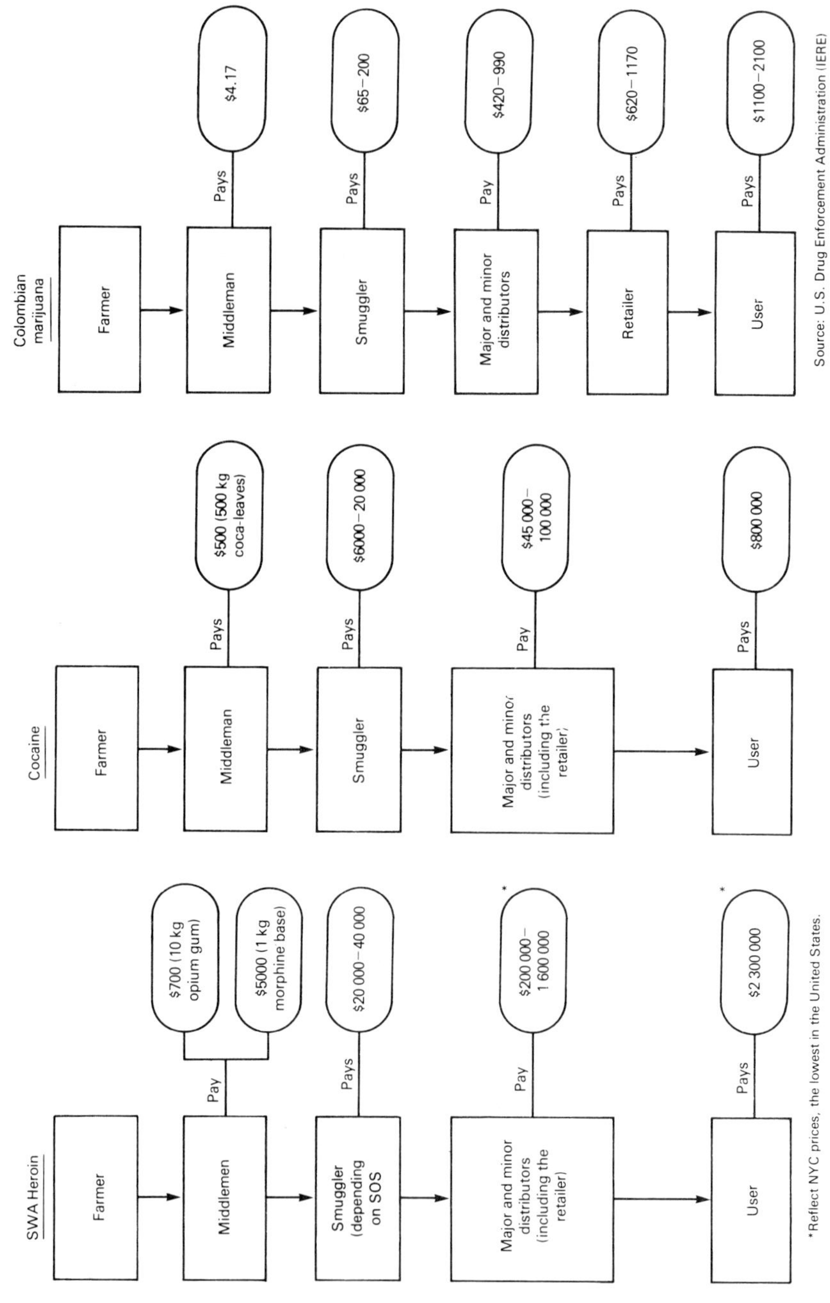

Figure 2.2 SWA heroin, cocaine and Colombian marijuana prices in 1979 (representative prices based on the equivalent of 1 kg pure substance). Source: US Drug Enforcement Administration (ICRE)

much the same type of distribution. Motivation to divert is obvious from the tremendous increase in prices paid by the user when compared with those paid by middlemen to the farmer. A kilogram of heroin, in 1979, brought US $700 to the farmer, but after processing was sold for US $2 300 000 at retail prices in the illegal street market.

It seems clear that in today's drug market economics plays the leading role. Blum *et al.* (1974, p. 62) describe the competition among interest groups on decision-making about how drugs are to be controlled in a society. Blum says, 'The competing domains are medicine and its associated basic sciences, those in the administration of justice, moral and logical thinkers, social scientists and social philosophers and drug consumers'. His dispassionate description may be a rational description of the negotiations through which a society in control of itself will go, when it has the time and perceives the need. Unfortunately, in the real world it is almost never an easy task and the rational solution may really be the rationalized one, given the requirements of particular circumstances.

The clash among interests is described in many ways. Unfortunately, these interests frequently lose sight of, or do not agree upon, the ultimate purposes, uses, controls, and limitations on drugs. Where the disagreements are fundamental, it is not the rational but the most powerful who generally prevail. For example, it is proven that alcohol causes many more deaths per year in those countries where it is legally sold than does heroin. Yet the political and social anxiety is greater over 3000 heroin-related deaths and 450 000 addicts in the United States, than for the 25 000 alcohol-related traffic deaths and the many thousands of other deaths each year medically identified as from alcoholism. Though drug-related crime is described and documented in detail, and it reveals that alcohol use is involved in many more crimes than other drug abuse, the power of the entrenched alcoholic beverage interests is such that demands for control are relatively ineffective.

This discussion is not meant to justify less effort in controlling illicit drugs. The ravages of opium and heroin abuse certainly should be prevented whenever they appear. The comparison is made to provide some illumination of the social decisions involved in eliminating drug problems when they become entrenched in the economic fabric of a society. Economics is at the root of the production of poppies in the golden triangle, in South-west Asia, Mexico, and elsewhere, in coca production in South America, in cannabis production throughout the world.

It is also the reason for production of legal drugs such as amphetamines, tranquillizers, antidepressants and other drugs. Where the economic and the socially approved coincide, there is a reasonable economic reward and appropriate use of drugs. Where there is a demand for the drug – legal or illegal – which outstrips legally approved supplies and is socially and legally disapproved, an illicit market can spring up which requires control if society is to preserve itself. The issue of morality inevitably arises in discussions of drug abuse. Blum *et al.*

(1974, p. 65) say that, 'Perhaps it is only when moral diversity and conflict, as well as heterogeneity of behaviour (pluralism) emerge that "objective" standards are called into play by which to shape and judge the laws. That secular scientific objectivity is itself, as the Kalants observe, a culture value and perhaps a culture phase.' There is an inevitable conflict between scientific objectivity and moral values in most societies. These are negotiated by the society's institutions. Where the issues are difficult to reconcile, problems continue. In today's world most societies are pluralist, and therefore require some kind of moral–social–scientific evaluation of legal controls.

Criteria are difficult to generalize in this field because of the variety of concerns. Nevertheless, the more important concerns are as follows:

(1) Might the result of changes in control be less desirable than the present circumstance? (This is a difficult question since political and social objectives often differ, and what may be good for society may not be acceptable to the political entities responsible such as crop substitution, eradication, legalization etc.)
(2) Is the control scheme consistent with other methods already accepted by the society or community?
(3) Can control be maintained by existing measures and control agencies performing more efficiently?
(4) Is control, if not possible with present resources, feasible if reasonable additional measures are taken?
(5) Is control a 'must' issue – that is, is it politically and/or socially essential regardless of the costs and other consequences?
(6) Will the controls be accepted by the society?
(7) What is the 'intensity' of opposition to additional controls, and does it balance with the demands for them? (This question may be phrased in many ways but the issue is frequently whether, once the controls are in place, will there be continuing problems, and will the added controls result in more or less social and political unrest.)
(8) Will added or reduced controls create problems in other areas, for example, too great a grant of power to administrative, enforcement, political, economic or social agencies?
(9) Will the changes in controls be seriously offensive to traditions, religious beliefs, or social institutions, to the extent that they will be a continuing source of conflict, and if so, what are the alternatives? Will controls merely change the source of the objections and changing pressure?
(10) Should the control changes be temporary or permanent, and should this be made clear in promulgating them?
(11) Will failure of control changes result in more serious problems than not instituting them, or taking other measures?
(12) Have alternatives to control measures been sufficiently considered, for example, will control 'institutionalize' the problem rather than resolve it?

(13) Is the control issue part of a larger problem which may be affected, and what problems might result?
(14) Is the part of the population to be controlled influential beyond their numbers, or conversely, are they relatively ineffectual politically and socially? (And will controls perhaps initiate undesirable action by such groups?)
(15) Can control proposals become so political that expedient rather than effective measures are chosen, and if so, should decisions be postponed or other alternatives chosen?
(16) Have the entities competing over the kinds of controls been identified by the decision-makers? Can there be negotiation, compromise or other reduction of conflict, or is the situation too far developed to be resolved by goodwill agreements?

These questions are not criteria, but aspects of the decision-making process at the policy level which should be considered before appropriate and knowledgeable decisions can be made. Of course, if the circumstances are such that there will be little or no conflict, and a law or regulation will resolve the problem, such considerations need not be a part of the decision-making process. Nevertheless, in most societies today there are serious disagreements over how controls on drugs are to be maintained or established. The interest of government at all levels is not the only one: pharmaceutical manufacturers, physicians and other health professionals, researchers, educators, retail sellers of drugs, and courts and law enforcement agencies all have an interest in controls on drugs. For some, the main concern will be financial; for others it will be a combination of professional, legal and ethical; while for still others it will be an ideological issue. And there is the general public which perceives only vaguely the need for and operation of controls but who are the object of concern of those who sell drugs, those who inveigh against them, and those who see the control issue as one that relates to freedom to choose. The moral–ideological issues become the most difficult to resolve, especially when freedom to abuse drugs and alcohol is at the expense of the children of those who have little interest or concern in abstractions. Most of these merely wish to raise their families and live in an environment less likely to force them to accept responsibility to control drugs, which they feel to be the responsibility of someone else.

The establishment of control, in the last analysis, requires a clear statement of objectives, administrative methodology, and expected results. There seem to be no great success stories in drugs and drug abuse control in today's chronicle of the problem. But what happens when there have been no efforts to control have caused most societies to continue to try.

PENALTIES

The spectrum of penalties for the production, distribution, possession and use of psychoactive substances is as broad as for any other crime, from forfeiture of goods or money, to imprisonment and death. The study of 153 countries by the US Department of State (Bureau of International Narcotics of Matters, 1979), though incomplete, revealed that of the 125 countries reported on, 55 do not distinguish between illegal activities involving narcotics and other prohibited substances (p. 4). A few (eight) have no penalties for possession of small amounts of cannabis, but most others provide for either a fine or imprisonment or both. However, none permit trafficking, and a third impose penalties varying from 10 years to death for cannabis offences.

There is insufficient space here for a full report of the study, but some highlights will be representative of the data. Ten countries allow possession of coca-leaf or cocaine for personal use, but as with cannabis, distribution, production and trafficking are prohibited. The laws are similar for the opium poppy and its derivatives. Of course, the judicial process varies widely, and where there is discretion, often the penalties actually given are not the maximums specified in the statutes.

The fact that legislation exists does not mean that it is, or can be, enforced effectively. In many countries today, there are epidemics of drug abuse, massive treatment programmes for addicts, medical administration of controlled substances for health maintenance requirements, and distribution through illegal channels.

Social and legal controls have similar characteristics and consequences in most societies. Where large numbers of the population are unwilling to obey the control, it is ineffective or very expensive to maintain. The question then becomes what accommodation can be developed between those who violate the law, those who administer it, and the society generally, who must support and finance administration and enforcement.

As can be seen from the international control scheme and the taxonomy described above, there are many levels of control, and many ways of achieving it. These become issues in a social conflict to be resolved by some form of consensus or acquiescence, and involve the following questions:

(1) Why should the substance be controlled?
(2) How, at what level, should it be controlled?
(3) Who is to control it – what agency, what formal or informal group or organization?
(4) What sanctions are appropriate – what are the reasonable relationships among the objectives, the individual offences and the sanctions?

The negotiation of these issues involves a number of factors including the type of offence – possession, distribution, production, trafficking, financing – as well as the type of substance, the status of the persons involved, the financial aspects, costs of enforcement, social costs, and the complexity of prosecution.

Thus far we have discussed in general terms the kinds of control mechanism available to control agencies within societies, governments and international organizations.

There are a multitude of public and social policy issues intertwined in legislation and control efforts. These involve not only local and national concerns but international political, economic and social structures and relationships. Only a brief discussion of some of the major issues is possible here. Important concerns are lack of intrinsic controls in individuals of their own appetites, desires and resultant behaviour as well as the need for controls and limitations on certain aspects of modern industrial activities.

OTHER RELATED CONCERNS

Public policy with regard to chemicals in industrial and commercial uses is a separate but related issue involving pure food laws, purity of water and air, controls on industrial wastes, radioactive substances, and chemicals used in agriculture and manufacturing. These substances, some of them highly toxic, are continuously ingested by breathing, eating or absorption. The role of chemicals in our society has expanded so explosively that in many cases no controls are possible until significant damage has occurred to the environment or individuals. Problems with nuclear fuel, hormones and antibiotics used in livestock feeding, industrial chemicals used in production or preparation of goods, and general air quality are but a few. These are mentioned to provide a perspective for discussion of substance-abuse issues which are merely a part of a much broader spectrum of concerns relating to ingestion of chemicals. Public education and formal instruction in schools appear to be inadequate in most countries, on the subjects of self-medication, health and hygiene, and environmental safety. As modern technology advances, the level of risk and danger to entire populations increases. Control of the production, distribution and use of chemicals for a variety of essential purposes seems to be inevitable. As the world population increases, international agreements will be necessary. The issues of regulation of air pollution, radioactive wastes, and pesticides even today make clear the complex kinds of future regulation and control issues which can arise.

GENERAL DISCUSSION OF CONTROL ISSUES

The legal control of psychoactive substances involves some measure of limitation on either access to and production of the substance itself, or controls on those who produce, or have, or seek access to, the substance. Thus, the controls are on the substance or the individual controlling the substance. The more complex the interrelationships among these two elements and the third, delivery from the source to the user, the more difficult control becomes.

Policy and legislation dealing with controls must take situations as they are and determine the possible alternatives and methodology for achieving the objectives of the policy and legislation, given the resources and power available. In countries such as Bolivia, Pakistan, Colombia, Iran, Thailand and others producing controlled substances, the system of production control is weak or non-existent. Efforts to control production have generally been ineffective, and movement of such drugs out of these countries has been relatively easy. In these countries drug control has a low priority. Resolving the production and transportation control problems in such countries would require diversion of scarce resources. Demands by so-called 'victim' countries – those to which drugs are shipped – for internal control are met with the response that if there were no market there would be no need for control, or requests for financial and technical assistance to the producers for crop substitution programmes or for enforcement activities such as spraying of illegal crops.

The United Nations is in fact orchestrating a modest effort to assist in world drug controls through the United Nations Fund for Drug Abuse Control, and the International Narcotics Control Board, which administers the two major treaties: the Single Convention on Narcotic Drugs of 1961 and the 1971 Convention on Psychotropic Substances.

The INCB is the successor to international drug control bodies established over the past half-century and has specific responsibilities (International Narcotics Control Board, 1980).

> Thus, on the one hand, the Board 'shall endeavour to limit the cultivation, production, manufacture and use of drugs to an adequate amount required for medicinal and scientific purposes and to ensure their availability for such purposes'. On the other hand, the Board shall endeavour 'to prevent illicit cultivation, production, and manufacture of, and illicit traffic in and use of, drugs'. In carrying out its responsibility the Board acts in cooperation with Governments and pursues continuing dialogues with them in order to further the aims of the treaties.

Clearly, a great deal of legislation is required for the regulation and control of the large number of psychoactive substances entering, leaving and being moved within most countries. For example a 1977 report to the President of the United States includes the following strategy components for a comprehensive policy review: 'international initiatives, domestic drug investigations, drug smuggling interdiction, regulation and compliance, and support programs such as intelligence, training, and science and technology' (Office of Drug Abuse Policy, Executive Office of the President, 1977, p. i).

The report identified several major problems in drug law enforcement which are similar to those in other developed nations:

(1) insufficient judicial resources and practices;
(2) inadequate supporting legislation;
(3) relative ambiguity in the policy implementation process;

(4) inadequate coordination and cooperation among government agencies involved in the illicit drug supply reduction activities;
(5) inadequate clarification of national priorities and the respective roles of state and local governments.

The problems of drug control require policy decisions based on both implicit and expressed societal objectives. In addition, the priorities for the expenditure of resources and manpower will determine levels of control. These considerations are generally dealt with at a level above the operational. That is, those who make policy, legislation and budget allocation decisions are not usually those who carry out the administration, regulation and control functions. The resources, mission, organization and function of the operational agencies theoretically are balanced against the perceived threat and need for control. The resources assigned are, unfortunately, not always consistent with the threat or the requirements of effective control, regulation and enforcement functions. A simple example illustrates the conflict between policy and practice. In the United States since the early 1900s laws in most states have required health education programmes on alcohol, drug and other substance abuse, and frequently abuse of tobacco as well. The training schools, however, because of other priorities have rarely provided adequate training and information to teachers, who then are ill-prepared to do the required instruction. In the 1960s when drug abuse became a national issue there was almost no accurate information on drugs which was widely available, and it has taken 15 years to develop the school programme to a level where in 1979 for the first time statistics on drug abuse by 17-year-olds have shown a slight decline from the year before (University of Michigan Institute for Social Research, 1980).

Examples of compromise in policy and resource allocation in treatment, law enforcement and public education are common. The cannabis issue does not need explanation here, since the amelioration of penalties for possession has been in part due to the lack of will to prosecute, lack of ability to enforce and courts to handle large numbers of offenders, and lack of ability of control mechanisms on the movement of cannabis across borders and within the countries involved. Heavy penalties in the law are largely ignored in many areas because of the realities of the situation.

The maintenance of opiate addicts rather than the enforcement of abstinence, controls on production of amphetamines and barbiturates, and alcohol rationing are common control measures when total prohibition is not feasible. The contradictions between providing government subsidies for tobacco production and an official antismoking campaign is obvious, yet both tobacco-growing and health are social priorities.

One of the most serious issues, and the most confusing, is the relationship of drugs to criminal activity. The polarization of this issue is most clear in the United States. In the 1930s policy-makers did not question the crime–drugs relationship very much. However, after the Second

World War it became a major issue because of legal definition of drug addiction as an illness rather than a crime in itself, and subsequently legislation was passed requiring different handling of users from possessors of illicit drugs. Use of a drug, the law said, was not a crime, only possession of it was illegal. The user was to be treated, not punished. The resultant confusion has still not been resolved. In the 1960s and 1970s research was done which was generalized to argue that although criminal activity increased after a person became addicted, addicts were not hardened criminals and were not responsible for non-drug-related crime. Research showed that at least some criminals were only incidentally addicts, but this was discounted by policy-makers and legislators, whose faith in the 'medical model' impelled them to believe that if addiction was 'cured', criminal activity would be reduced. And in so far as the treatment facilities exercised control of the addicts, criminal activity did in fact decrease.

What was not well-understood, however, was that there is no absolute cause-and-effect relationship between addiction and criminal activity. Either may be a cause or an effect. A study done in 1974 by the US Law Enforcement Assistance Administration (LEAA) (Barton, 1974) found that an estimated 61% of the 191 400 inmates of state correctional facilities had used drugs such as heroin, methadone, cocaine, marijuana, amphetamines or barbiturates at some point in their lives without a doctor's prescription. In addition, the study found that six out of every ten inmates had been under the influence of drugs or alcohol at the time of the offences which caused their present imprisonment.

From the more conservative perspective of the 1980s, crime and drugs are again being examined. A recent study (Ball *et al.*, 1980) found that a random sample of 243 addicts from the streets of a large US city admitted to committing 473 738 offences over an 11-year period. This is consistent with the previously cited study of state prison inmates done in 1974 (Barton, 1974), and a follow-up study by LEAA done in 1978. This study showed that 55% of prisoners admitted to being under the influence of drugs or alcohol while committing the crime for which they were imprisoned. It is clear that drugs and crime are related more closely than was believed by policy-makers in the 1960s. However, the protests of law enforcement officers went largely unheard. Even addicts themselves said that to eliminate the two problems they needed to be dealt with separately. Ex-addicts and 'street people' who founded treatment programmes are almost unanimous in saying that the individual's crime needs punishment and his addiction needs treatment. And slowly this dual approach has been accepted. Yet the problem of drug-related crime remains as long as drug trafficking cannot be controlled. Some authorities call for dealing with the 'career criminal' who may use drugs but would be a criminal whether or not he/she used them. This would control the most vicious criminals, but would not by itself solve the problem of crime committed by addicts. The Ball *et al.* (1980) study showed that criminal activity increased when the individual was addicted and dropped when he or she was drug-free. Control of the supply of drugs to the level of almost complete unavailability in an area or community is possible, and will probably be necessary to eliminate drug-related crime. In the early 1970s a few communities focused upon prosecution of drug addicts themselves, and indeed were successful in moving the addicts out of the community. However, the availability of drugs elsewhere merely relocated the drug–crime problem. Nevertheless, crime did decrease in those communities. The lessons here are far from clear, but they do point to the need for greater controls on drug users themselves than have been believed necessary by legislators and policy-makers. The 'medical model' may be a means of reducing addiction, but its curative powers do not reach as far as to permanently reduce crime. The control exercised over addicts in treatment is an important factor in crime reduction, however, as is the fact that money to purchase drugs is no longer needed.

Two factors seem significant here: control of the addict appears to reduce criminal activity by addicts, and control of drug availability can control the addict. Thus, either providing the addict with drugs, or preventing access to the drug can reduce crime by those persons. The balance between these two kinds of control is dictated by policy-makers in their allocation of resources and establishment of priorities. In the United States it costs between $3000 and $5000 per year per addict for treatment in an outpatient clinic. Law enforcement costs are not easily estimated. However, the costs of crime related to drug addiction is estimated in the billions of dollars each year in the United States. A cost–benefit ratio between treatment and control measures should be developed for each country to determine which policy will be most effective for the monetary expenditure. The social costs must, of course, also be included, and may override economic considerations in some instances. As we shall see below, it may be possible to finance law enforcement efforts from the activities of the enforcement agencies themselves and so keep the costs of control proportional to the amount of criminal activity. But care must be taken to avoid a symbiotic relationship where addiction, treatment, enforcement and drug dealing interact to perpetuate a drug abuse 'industry'. Public education is the means of breaking this interactive chain.

REGULATION OF LEGALLY PRODUCED DRUGS

Professional control and monopoly of legally produced and dispensed drugs has become increasingly important as new mood-altering drugs such as meprobamate, glutethimide, methaqualone, apart from hundreds of others, have been marketed over the past 25 years. The control of production and promotion of such drugs has become increasingly important, and, as these synthetics proliferate, increasingly difficult. Such drugs rarely are disease-specific or used in the treatment of physiological illness. Rather they are of great value in reducing psychological symptoms when properly prescribed.

The potential for abuse is extremely high, however. Such drugs are frequently misprescribed by busy physicians, diverted by drug handlers, or illegally manufactured in unlicensed laboratories.

The report of the International Narcotics Control Board (1980) strongly addresses this issue:

> The Board considers it timely to make the overall observation that effective international control of psychoactive substances is proving more complex than was originally foreseen because of the large number of such substances, their extensive use in medical practice, their rapidly developing non-medical uses, and the great potential for clandestine manufacture of certain of them. Moreover, the international control system for psychotropic substances, unlike that for narcotic drugs, does not set forth arrangements for establishing anticipated medical and scientific requirements against which manufacturing output can be matched. This makes it difficult to monitor supply and demand effectively, both nationally and worldwide. Substantial licit overproduction already appears to exist in the case of amphetamines, posing potential risks for diversion, misuse and abuse. Besides manufacturing statistics furnished to the Board may not be provided by all countries and therefore cannot be presumed to constitute total manufacture.

The report also points out that substantial amounts of abused substances are diverted from legal manufacture and trade and that precursors are readily available for illegal manufacturing. It also says that the growing abuse of psychotropic substances is of great concern and that the control situation is similar to that which existed with opiates in the 1920s and early 1930s for legal production of opiates. The differences are that psychotropics are much more numerous and widely used and traded internationally through numerous transactions. Statistics available to the Board reveal substantial discrepancies in amphetamines and methaqualone between medical need and manufacture. In countries where controls on manufacture have been imposed, manufacture and importation have been enormously reduced. In the United States, for example, amphetamine manufacturing has been reduced by 97% since the initiation of production quotas in 1973.

Reasonable controls can be defined by many factors. Where there is little diversion of drugs to non-addict users, minimal controls are sufficient. In today's world, unfortunately, the potential for abuse problems exists almost everywhere. That is why the discussion of control in this chapter emphasizes controls necessary to reduce, prevent or deter illicit traffic and abuse. In a world where there was little abuse, control legislation would be confined to the dusty shelves of legal libraries.

POLICY GUIDELINES

Those who set policy and propose legislation and regulations to make them relevant and effective must understand the nature of drug control and the unique aspects of drug trafficking – from producer through distributor and seller to the user. Understanding by itself, however, is insufficient. Legislation on drug control requires flexibility in dealing with the complex interrelationships of the kinds of substances, production, trafficking, habituated users, legal and illegal distribution channels, media, and public opinion.

Where laws and regulations do not fit the circumstances, enforcement is difficult or impossible. Easy bail and low sentencing practices of many courts in the United States are an example which shows how criminals who are apprehended by enforcement agencies escape appropriate punishment. Major criminals with access to millions of dollars in cash are freed on bond by the courts; they then forfeit the bond, which is a small fraction of the profits of their illegal activity, and escape the country. This encourages others to enter trafficking, and drug laws no longer remain an effective deterrent. Deterrence is an essential aspect of control; where it is impossible to enforce laws effectively, their failure reveals the weakness of the authority and thus the futility of the law itself.

Decisions must be made on alternative measures for control and enforcement to assure the effectiveness of the legal sanction which is the expression of the will of the society. Alternative measures to enforcement are essential to permit flexibility in control efforts. The limitations of a control policy based solely on apprehension of drug sellers must be recognized, and public education and information utilized to assist in sharing responsibility with other social institutions such as the educational system, social agencies and responsible public officials. The health and education professions have a responsibility in social control which cannot be abdicated without serious consequences.

A society which seeks to preserve and perpetuate itself must have the ability to control appropriately the individuals within it, who therefore comprise it. When a society no longer has the will or the lead time to marshal its political, economic or social organization and resources within existing controls to deal with a problem, then its options become very limited. The time to make control decisions is when the society, through its institutions, still has the opportunity to choose from among alternatives that are not destructive of its basic institutions. The choice of whether to control importation and production of drugs or to apprehend drug addicts may not present itself in a clear-cut fashion. But clearly the former is more cost-effective, easier to administer, and involves fewer social consequences. In spite of this, many societies prefer to endure the expense of treating drug addicts rather than take the necessary measures to control illicit sales, or provide for long-term education on health, safety, and self-medication. This may be because present legislation does not permit effective control, or because of financing problems – control agencies would require too much additional funding. Alternatively the emotional desire to find a 'humane' solution may influence decision-makers who find it easier to deal with the educated 'health professional' than with the tough-minded 'law enforcement professional'. There are other easily deduced reasons for delaying decisions. This is not to say that the decisions themselves are easy. However, when they are not taken the opportunity to choose is often lost, and then both kinds of measures – increased health care and increased control measures – and their respective costs, become necessary. In the United States, the costs to the federal budget alone are about $700 million per year. This is, significantly, approximately equally divided between control (enforcement and regulation) and non-control measures (treatment, research, education).

The drug problem has the potential of weakening the fabric of society – family relationships, responsible citizenship, productive occupations. Where these are weakened, other factors, external and internal, may combine with drug and alcohol abuse to seriously wound the society.

Controls are available and can be used when a society is aware of the threat and recognizes the need to choose from among the reasonable options those which are most effective and most realistic. But the primary requirements are that the society or community

(1) recognizes the danger and the need for control; and
(2) has the will to do what is necessary,
   (a) to allocate sufficient resources to deal with the problem, and
   (b) to control what needs to be controlled in the circumstances, illicit and legal production, the legal marketplace, the illicit dealer, the user, or a combination of these.

Decisions on appropriate combinations of these factors – drug, user, seller – can be made with the support of the public and its active co-operation, if that support is marshalled in appropriate ways within the power of the social and political leadership.

The less official control that exists in a society, the more difficult it is to marshal such support. In some nations the social institutions – church, home, school, community leadership – are the leaders of and makers of public opinion. In countries where social unrest, heterogeneity of values, an undisciplined media, political instability, or lack of social controls exist, controls of any kind may be unsuccessful.

The United States provides an excellent example of the kinds of problems that exist in a nation where political control is stable, but social control often depends upon a consensus and the influence of the media. Iran, on the other hand, is an example of weak political control but strong social (in this case religious) control. Both countries have serious drug problems – cannabis and synthetic drugs in the United States and opiates in Iran. But epidemics of drug abuse have stricken such homogeneous countries as Japan (amphetamines), Sweden and other Scandinavian countries (amphetamines and alcohol), Britain (cannabis and alcohol), Germany (heroin), and the Netherlands (cannabis). Russia, another heterogeneous country, has a severe alcohol problem, despite strong political control.

Drug abuse cannot be barred by national boundaries in the modern world. The need for control exists in varying ways in almost every country for some mood-altering substance. The question is, what will work?

It is clear that in the short-term certain measures can succeed: for example, stringent laws and firm enforcement by police against drug *users and dealers*. Where sufficient resources are brought to bear, the using and dealing population is small enough, and the courts are willing to provide adequate punishment, enforcement efforts *can* work. This has been shown where the penalties are

(1) known by the potential offenders;
(2) known to the public to be applied to actual offenders;
(3) administered fairly and openly to all offenders;
(4) and appropriate to the offences.

It is the *reality* of punishment which is the deterrent, where the consequences of prosecution of an offence are understood by the persons involved. Deterrence, however, involves acquiescence by the overwhelming majority of the population. Where this is lacking, stringent laws alone will not work. Civil disobedience exists in almost every society and the political sanctions are inadequate to deal with it in the long term, although it may be somewhat controllable in the short term.

Therefore, in the long view, the goal of a society must be acquiescence of citizens to controls and limitations, while the controls can still be exercised on the passive majority of the population, who may care very little or not at all about abusing drugs. When a social movement such as drug abuse and experimentation starts, whether it is stimulated by easy drug availability (as in many developing countries), media sensationalizing (as in developed countries), or a combination of these and the example of youth groups who interact through universities, travel, or rock music, it can be controlled at the outset by limiting drug availability, at least to some extent. But as the number of users increases, the momentum of demand and pressures on supply–control increase until existing controls on supplies of the drug of choice are inadequate. The level of control may then focus on the seller, but where sellers are numerous (they may also be users who are financing their need for the drug) control becomes difficult.

AN ECONOMIC SOLUTION

The economic aspects of drug dealing may be the most vulnerable in the illicit drug markets. Where there is little or no profit, sellers of illicit drugs are less numerous and less imaginative. Where the economic risks are high – loss of goods, money, possessions – dealers will avoid them. Where the economic costs to the user is high, he will be to some degree deterred from using drugs. However, where supplies are available, even when the cost is high, there will be some users willing to purchase once they have become dependent upon the substance as part of their lifestyles.

Still, increasing the costs to the seller and the user is an effective control mechanism because it discourages *recruitment* of new users who are not yet habituated by psychological, physical or environmental dependence on the drug. Thus, the research finding that control of drugs in a community is a function of the availability of all drugs abused is confirmed. Tight controls make the seller cautious about whom he sells to, thus reducing new users.

At present, most costs of control and enforcement have been absorbed by governments and responsible agencies. Effective economic principles would dictate that controls on drugs support themselves. To some extent this is the case with alcohol in many countries, where taxes are high. Legally produced drugs for medical purposes are taxed both directly and indirectly. There are licensing fees and direct taxes, but there are also the 'fees' paid by patients to physicians and pharmacists who dispense the drugs. These financial controls are in many cases sufficient to limit abuse to a small proportion of the total use.

The controls on alcohol are certainly complex and difficult to analyse, but it is clear that without them there would be even more abuse than there is now. Countries with strong laws against driving while intoxicated have reduced social costs significantly, for example. Where there are tobacco controls, taxes often support the control effort. Unfortunately, social acceptance of tobacco use complicates newly required health controls. This is similar to the control problem for psychotropic substances with valid medical uses. The user may legally obtain the substance – amphetamine, barbiturate, tranquillizer, etc. – but still abuse it. Control must then be on the seller/dispenser, where distribution can be controlled, or on both producer and seller/dispenser where production also is controllable.

Financial controls on drug trafficking can be effected in two ways. First, by identifying the financial assets of drug traffickers and seizing them after they have been accumulated. This is possible, as experience during alcohol prohibition in the United States in the 1930s showed. It does not, however, deal with the immediate problem. That is, the drugs have already been sold and used.

The second method of financial control expropriates the funds destined for the major trafficker before they reach him. The purchaser/user and small-amount seller, are the sources of the millions which find their way into the bank accounts of drug-trafficking financiers. To make it more difficult for such funds to accumulate, fines, forfeiture of property, legal judgments, seizure of assets can be levied on possessors of any amount of a substance. Where these levies are sufficiently high, the user cannot afford to continue use and so drops out of the market. Of course, where the user is a confirmed drug addict, he or she will attempt to use other drugs or turn to criminal activity to obtain money to buy the drugs. However, treatment and compulsory rehabilitation are now part of most drug control efforts, and a levy on users can finance that treatment.

There are certain problems in designing a system of controls to meet the varying needs of a society to control the elements in its drug problem – production, distribution, seller, user. Some countries, such as the United States, are reluctant to expend the resources necessary to control the problem, having other higher-priority problems. However if the costs can be borne by the trafficker rather than the public treasury, there may be greater motivation to take the appropriate measures. For example, until 1970, the United States had in effect a tax of $100 per ounce on marijuana. This tax was collected by the Internal Revenue Service from any person in possession of cannabis, even though the drug was illegal. Court decisions and a comprehensive revision of the US drug laws eliminated this tax. However, taxation is still a valid method of revenue collection and might well be used in local law enforcement efforts. If such a tax would support the drug control effort, it would be enthusiastically accepted by the citizen who has fears for his children's involvement in drugs. In some countries, a bounty system for customs and other seizures, though sometimes susceptible to corruption, is already in place. Forfeiture and tax legislation aimed at highly abused drugs is a logical step towards placing the economic burden of drug control on those who make necessary a high level of control – illicit sellers and users.

Approaching drug abuse from the economic aspects and attempting to establish a system whereby the drug user, seller and trafficker become the source of support for the enforcement, treatment, rehabilitation and education programmes they make necessary may be viable and should be attempted. A revenue-sharing procedure, by which local enforcement agencies are financially motivated to enforce the drug laws would, of course, be an important aspect of such a system.

Drug control measures, as we have seen, must vary with the problem as perceived by the society in which it exists. Anticipation, careful planning, clearly established objectives, adequate financial support, effective utilization of manpower, high-level policy support, and a well-coordinated control system – from production through distribution to the user – these are the essentials. But they are still not sufficient. The will of society and public acceptance of the need to control are necessary for controls to succeed.

SOCIAL EDUCATION NEEDS

In the longest term, extrinsic controls are not the most efficient method of dealing with social problems. When one considers that a society renews itself through birth and death over a span of two generations, it is easily understood that measures that make possible the elimination of controls for antisocial behaviour are the most desirable. Those countries which pride themselves on fostering freedom and independence among their citizens are sometimes reluctant to examine their educational systems to determine how effectively they inculcate the mores, taboos, ethics and principles of social behaviour which make their society what it is. But in fact any country which neglects its educational system and which builds into it the seeds of doubt about the society's values opens itself to damage. Education on the entire topic of substance abuse, self-medication and the effects of chemicals on the individual and society should be part of any modern social education system throughout life.

This is not to say that all education must be conditioning, or in the popular phrase, 'brainwashing'. Nevertheless, a basic faith is necessary in the traditional values preserved by a society in its institutions, its beliefs, its literature, its folkways, its manners, its traditions and its conscience. Without that common core of shared, accepted and defended ideas, it cannot survive for long nor develop and grow. The alternative is of course to degenerate. Socially destructive loss of self-control, pursuit of self-indulgence, loss of self-respect, unwillingness to postpone gratification, inability to sacrifice for the greater good, disregard of ethical and legal constraints, these consequences of drug abuse and drug dependence in too many of today's youth are a grave warning.

CONCLUSIONS

The subject of drug control legislation has been described in many ways and from many perspectives. It has been impossible to deal comprehensively with even a single important issue in this brief chapter. The materials presented here are necessarily in the nature of generalizations drawn from materials themselves often generalized and summarized. The necessary data and logical analyses to make the chapter fully self-contained can of course be found in other material, and, though the conclusions and analyses are the writer's own, there is ample data to support them.

Present drug control and regulation policies in many countries are not equal to the requirements for drug control. There has been a failure of the 'medical model' for control of drug abuse through treatment alone because it is too often not accompanied by other necessary controls. The facts reveal that the failure is often due to overdependence on a single measure. The roles of communication, education, social institutions, and individuals in key 'gatekeeper' positions are poorly defined, and their responsibilities are not clear. The movement and destinations of psychoactive substances, legal and illegal, is badly documented or not recorded at all because of limitations of resources for control.

Drug control legislation has generally developed as a *response* to an existing and growing problem rather than in anticipation of problems. These 'after-the-fact' efforts merely acknowledge and underline, in many instances, the problem which the legislation is designed to control. For example, reduction of the penalties for possession of small amounts of cannabis has occurred in many places, after it was clear that the laws controlling cannabis were being ignored by both citizens and enforcement agencies, and cases were being dismissed by courts. The result was, predictably, increased availability and use.

This discussion has been intended to stimulate thought about the need for clarity and coherence in social policy and legislation on drug control. It suggests that the most effective controls have been and generally still are in the economic areas. The tax collector has traditionally been the most effective enforcement agent, and the most persistent. It is not argued here that the policies and legislation of the past are necessarily wrong. Rather that they may be ineffective because they are not supported sufficiently by the political, financial, administrative and social structures in a community or political entity. If the will to resolve the situation is not there, or if it is but there are no means by which that will can be expressed and its purposes carried out, then the problem remains.

It may be that comprehensive drug control, like Christianity, to quote G. K. Chesterton, has not failed, it has not really been tried. The measures proposed have been many, but they focus on symptoms and effects for the most part, or are too general to be identified as successful or unsuccessful, as in such programmes as 'alternatives' to drug abuse. These may work, but should be provided in any case, whether drug abuse exists or not. Young people *should* be interested in the arts, sports, social activities and helping others not because it keeps them from abusing drugs, but because these are constructive pursuits. The direct measures – treatment, apprehension and arrest, imprisonment, and compulsory education – are reactive palliatives. Prevention and deterrence are proactive measures, but are ineffective as presently administered in most societies. In relatively permissive ones, they may be the only feasible ones, given the minimal resources provided by policy and legislation. But strong repressive measures, if sanctioned by the society, *do* work. Yet the cost is high if drugs are easily obtained.

Measures to legalize cannabis, or as in the United States, 'decriminalize' it (provide minor penalties short of imprisonment), have been proposed to solve the problem by pretending it no longer is a problem. Yet proponents have never been able to reconcile a policy which discourages abuse of a psychoactive substance – cannabis – with making it more easily available. The same contradictions exist with respect to alcohol and tobacco. A clear policy statement may exist, but often the administrative procedures and responsibility for carrying them out become diffuse, when conflicting interests are involved.

The spectrum of possible measures for drug control are clearly described in the literature. Clear objectives and reasonable policies may be expressed in some legislation and in international agreements for specific issues. The difficulties arise because of problems in coordination of the complexities in basic elements in the drug equation: drug, producer, distributor-seller, and user. How should they be controlled, in what balance and by what means, by whom and in what measure?

Where the policy issues can be resolved, legislation can be drawn which will conform to the policy. The realistic application of that legislation must involve compromise, but it must, at bottom, permit sufficient resources to be used to obtain acquiescence of the population. This is the dilemma. It is our thesis that control measures which do not unduly challenge beliefs, but which focus on the economic and practical concerns of ordinary persons, are likely to be the most effective. Where immediate impact on one's purse is felt, there is likely to be a change in behaviour.

The drug abuse issue, it is clear, has often been confused by the pseudo-philosophical meanderings of some whose facility and cleverness in semantics has obscured the need for a rational public policy. Drunkenness and loss of self-control, whether induced by alcohol or other intoxicating substances has never been accepted by any society except when described in mystical terms, or as a recreational or religious interlude in otherwise earnest social pursuits. When described in practical terms, the values of health, self-control, avoidance of psychological or physiological dependence are essential universal social and personal objectives.

This discussion has sought to restore practical and real, as opposed to pseudo-intellectual and mystical-philosophical perspectives to a problem too long obscured by sensation-seeking professional as well as non-professional groups and individuals with access to print and electronic media. More than one thoughtful expert in the field has identified the media and their allies – health and social scientists who lack a sense of perspective and social responsibility – as the initiators of the present world epidemic. To attribute such power to anyone is an admission of the weakness of the institutions which must bear the burden of counter-education and restoration of the society in which the conflict exists. Yet there is no question as to the power of mass media to inflict terrible damage to a society when it behaves irresponsibly. When the media behave responsibly, it is an equally powerful force for good. Unfortunately, it cannot undo all the evil it may be used to promote.

The naive, youthful, drug culture of the 1960s has passed. There is some indication that the hysteria about drugs, and the mystique given to it by the media, have begun to dissipate. Yet there remains the destructive force of the counter-culture's most insidious weapon – drug abuse. But now it is driven by the economic engine of illicit profit, not intellectual or political adventurism and irresponsibility. As world societies seek to renew themselves the legacy of the mindless pursuit of pleasure stimulated by drug-use advocates of the 1960s still remains to be dealt with by responsible societies in today's world.

REFERENCES

Ball, J. C., Rosen, L., Flueck, J. H. and Nurco, D. N. (1980). *The Criminality of Heroin Addicts When Addicted and When Off Opiates.* Paper presented to the International Congress on Alcoholism and Drug Dependence Level (ICAA) Medellin, Colombia, 3–6 December

Barton, W. A. (1980). *Drug Abuse History and Criminality of Inmates of Local Jails: Result of the 1978 LEAA Survey of Inmates of Local Jails in the United States*, (Washington, DC: US Drug Enforcement Administration)

Blum, R. H. and Bovet, D., Moore, J. *et al.* (1974). *Controlling Drugs: International Handbook for Psychoactive Drug Classification*, prepared by Jonathan Wolfe. (San Francisco: Jossey-Bass Publishers)

Bureau of International Narcotics of Matters. (1979). *The Global Legal Framework for Narcotics and Prohibitive Substances.* (Washington, DC: US Department of State)
Bureau of Narcotics and Dangerous Drugs. (1972). *A Study of International Control of Narcotics and Dangerous Drugs*, SCID-TR-5 (Vol. 1) (Washington, DC: US Department of Justice)
International Narcotics Control Board. (1980). *Report of the International Narcotic Control Board for 1980.* (New York: United Nations)
Office of Drug Abuse Policy, Executive Office of the President (1977). *Supply Control: Drug Law Enforcement and Interagency Review.* (Washington, DC)
University of Michigan Institute for Social Research. (1980). *Drugs and the Nation's High School Students. Five Year National Trends.* (Washington, DC: National Institute on Drug Abuse, US Department of Health and Human Services)

FURTHER READING

Annual Report on the Federal Drug Program. (1980). (Washington, DC: Executive Office of the President of the United States)
Austin, G. A. (1978). *Perspectives on the History of Psychoactive Substance Abuse.* (Washington, DC: US Department of HEW, National Institute on Drug Abuse)
Barton, W. I. (1980). Drug histories and criminality: survey of inmates of state correctional facilities, January, 1974. *Int. J. Addict.*, **15(2)**, 233
Brill, H. (1981). The new semantics of drug abuse. *Drug Abuse in the Modern World.* (New York: Pergamon Press)
Comptroller General Report to the Congress of the United States. (1979). *Gains Made in Controlling Illegal Drugs, Yet the Drug Trade Flourishes.* (Washington, DC: US General Accounting Office)
Inciardi, J. A. and Chambers, C. D. (1974). *Drugs and the Criminal Justice System.* (Beverly Hills, CA: Sage Publications)
Kay, D. A. (1976). *The International Regulation of Pharmaceutical Drugs.* The American Society of International Law. Studies in Transnational Legal Policy. No. 14. (Washington, DC)
National Institute on Drug Abuse. (1978). *International Drug Use.* Research Issues No. 23. (Washington, DC: US Department of Health, Education and Welfare)
National Narcotics Intelligence Consumers Committee. (1980). *Narcotics Intelligence Estimate; The Supply of Drugs to the U.S. Illicit Market From Foreign and Domestic Sources in 1979 (with Projections for 1980–83).* (Washington, DC)

3

British experience in the management of opiate dependence

H. B. Spear

DEVELOPMENT OF HEROIN ADDICTION IN THE UNITED KINGDOM

After almost a decade in which it seemed that the explosion of heroin abuse in the 1960s had been successfully contained, the numbers of new heroin addicts coming to notice in the United Kingdom are again rising and there is evidence of a substantial growing and well-organized criminal black market in the drug. Although the traditional sources of supply for the British opiate abuser, thefts from legitimate stocks in wholesale warehouses, hospitals, retail pharmacies, etc., and over-generous prescribing, are still relevant, illicit importation of heroin from South-east and South-west Asia and the Middle East provides the main initial source of supply for this new generation of abusers. The availability on the British market of appreciable quantities of illicit heroin represents a fundamental change in the character of the British opiate black market, which since the emergence of the heroin subculture in the early 1950s (Spear, 1969), had depended on the addict/pusher selling that part of his prescribed supply which was surplus to his immediate requirements, rather than on the non-addicted/pusher whose motives for selling heroin were entirely financial.

Just as the increase in heroin addiction in the 1960s was seen as a breakdown in the so-called 'British system', under which it was perfectly legal for an addict to receive supplies of drugs from a doctor, so the emergence of a criminal black market has been seen (Fazey, 1979) as an inevitable consequence of the current prescribing (or non-prescribing) policies of the treatment clinics which were established in 1967–68 following the second report of the Interdepartmental

Committee on Drug Addiction (Brain Committee, 1965). While some evidence can be adduced in support of both these points of view it would be wrong to interpret changes in the pattern of opiate dependence in the United Kingdom entirely in terms of availability of supplies of drugs.

Since the first Dangerous Drugs Regulations of 1921 the only limitation on a doctor's right to prescribe and supply morphine and heroin had been that his prescribing was to be 'for the exercise of his profession or employment', yet it was not until the early 1950s when the newly emerged group of hedonistic heroin addicts began to seek out successfully those doctors who, for a variety of reasons or motives, could be induced to prescribe heroin in liberal amounts, that this virtually unfettered right was seriously exploited. Clearly some complex social processes had occurred to create a demand for heroin where none had existed for the previous 30 years. Similarly, the current explosion of interest in heroin has occurred some 10 years after the treatment centres came into existence, and is undoubtedly linked to significant changes in social attitudes to this drug over the last few years. Whereas the 'alternative society' of the 1960s, while favouring the use of cannabis, drew the line at the use of heroin, there is now a disturbing acceptance by a wide section of society of heroin as a recreational drug. This trend has serious implications for British drug control policy which for the past 60 years has been based on the tenet that the addict is a sick person who needs medical treatment, too rigid an acceptance of which has undoubtedly contributed to some of the difficulties facing the country today.

OPIATE DEPENDENCE AND THE ROLLESTON COMMITTEE

The British experience of the management of opiate dependence can be conveniently reviewed in three distinct phases; the period from the establishment of the central philosophy of the 'British approach' by the Departmental Committee on Morphine and Heroin Addiction in 1926 (Rolleston Committee, 1926) until the end of the Second World War; from the emergence of a new proselytising group of heroin addicts in 1951 to the implementation of the recommendations of the second Brain Committee in 1968 and from then to the present time.

The first two periods have been the subject of detailed analysis by Bean and others (Bean, 1974; Judson, 1974; Spear, 1975) and require little further detailed discussion here, but it is nevertheless important to remember the reasons why the Rolleston and two Brain Committee enquiries were set up and the background against which each was conducted.

The Rolleston Committee was appointed in 1924 essentially to assist the Home Office, as the department responsible for carrying out Parliament's intentions as expressed in the Dangerous Drugs Act of 1920 and the Dangerous Drugs Regulations of 1921, in ensuring that the uses of such drugs should be confined to those necessary for the purposes of *bona fide* medical treatment. Following the passage of this legislation it became apparent that exceptionally large amounts of drugs had been or were being supplied to some doctors, or to individual patients on doctors' prescriptions, in circumstances where the drugs were clearly not part of the medical treatment of some organic disease but were simply to enable persons who had become addicted to satisfy their craving. The Committee's advice on the difficult question of whether or not the supply of drugs to such individuals constituted *bona fide* medical treatment was to form the cornerstone of British drug policy for the next 50 years. This advice was based on the assessment that addiction to morphine and heroin was not only rare but was diminishing, largely as a result of the operation of the new legislation, and that addiction was to be found most frequently amongst those who had previously had the drug in the course of medical treatment, persons engaged in occupations 'which entail much nervous and mental strain' or those, who by reason of their occupation or otherwise, had ready access to the drugs. Cases of addiction resulting from 'mere curiosity or search for pleasurable sensations' were exceptional and were expected to become less prevalent through the operation of the restrictions on supply imposed by the new legislation, but perhaps the most telling evidence that the Committee were dealing with a situation totally different from that of the 1980s is the statement that:

> Although sources of illegitimate supply exist, it appears that those who might, in other circumstances, have obtained the drugs from non-medical sources are usually lacking in the determination and ingenuity necessary for overcoming the obstacles which the law now places in their way.

While the Rolleston Committee could be criticized by anyone familiar with today's addicts for this comfortable view of some of society's most manipulative and resourceful individuals, their vision in providing for the policing of their main recommendations, by means of a medical tribunal, which could advise the Home Secretary whether or not there were sufficient medical grounds for the administration or supply of drugs by a doctor, could not. If there were no such grounds the Home Secretary could, on the tribunal's recommendations, prohibit the doctor from obtaining, possessing or supplying controlled drugs. In making this proposal, which is of major importance in the light of subsequent events, the Committee commented:

> We consider, therefore, that a Medical Tribunal constituted on the lines suggested above would afford valuable assistance to the Home Office in securing that possession and supply of the drugs by medical practitioners was restricted to that required for legitimate medical purposes, and would enable the Department to deal effectively and in a manner satisfactory to the medical profession, with a case in which there were strong grounds for believing that a doctor was administering drugs for illegitimate purposes either to himself or to others.

Provision for the establishment of such tribunals was made in the Dangerous Drugs Regulations of 1926 but the procedure was never invoked. The reasons for this are not now clear but seem likely to have been the lack of suitable cases for reference. From 1926 until the end of the Second World War there were very few recorded examples of the indiscriminate prescribing which was to attract such attention in the 1960s and those addict doctors, whom the Rolleston Committee also had in mind when making their recommendation, could usually be dealt with by other means. Although unused, the tribunal provisions remained in the Regulations until 1953 when they were omitted pending agreement with the medical profession about new rules of procedure. Unfortunately this was to prove a very costly omission because at the very time the rules of procedure were being renegotiated the urgent need for some machinery to deal with excessive prescribing became apparent. Two further misfortunes were also to overtake the restoration of the tribunal procedure. The first of these was the appointment of the Franks Committee on Tribunals (1957) which meant a delay of 4 years before the way was clear to restore the tribunal machinery; but the second, and far more serious, in the light of subsequent events, was the recommendation of the first report of the Interdepartmental Committee on Drug Addiction (Brain Committee, 1961) that 'the Home Secretary should not establish medical tribunals to investigate the grounds for recommending him to withdraw a doctor's authority to possess and supply dangerous drugs'.

THE BRAIN COMMITTEE'S RECOMMENDATIONS, AND AFTER

For this recommendation alone the first Brain Committee (1961) must stand accused of a lack of appreciation of the changes which were then occurring in the British opiate abuse scene and for not having the depth of vision of their predecessors in 1926. The Committee were impressed that 'the right of doctors in Great Britain to continue at their own professional discretion the provision of dangerous drugs to known addicts has not contributed to any increase in the total number of patients receiving regular supplies in this way'. Yet at the very time of the Committee's enquiry the spread of heroin addiction amongst young persons in London was being fuelled by medical prescriptions, a situation which had first been documented in the Home Office in 1955 and had been one of the reasons for the Home Office suggestion that the time was opportune for a review of the advice offered by the Rolleston Committee in 1926. Apart from believing that there was then, and in the foreseeable future, no need for a tribunal procedure, the Committee also saw considerable difficulties in setting up such machinery. Thus, they saw there would be need for power to take evidence on oath, addict witnesses would be notoriously unreliable and there would be conflicting medical opinion which would make it difficult to decide what constituted 'sufficient medical grounds' for the issue of a prescription to an addict. As will be seen later, the operation of the tribunals established under the Misuse of Drugs Act 1971 has shown that these fears were grossly overexaggerated.

The practical consequence of this recommendation was that for the next 12 years until tribunals were reinstituted by the Misuse of Drugs (Tribunal) Regulations in 1973 the Home Office had no effective means other than remonstration of dealing with any doctor whose prescribing to addicts gave rise to concern. (Brain, (1961) had 'strongly condemned' prescribing 'without providing adequate medical supervision, without making any determined effort at withdrawal and, notably, without seeking another medical opinion' but had not seen fit to provide machinery for satisfactorily terminating such action.) It was clear from a little known 'test case' in 1955 that the Courts were unlikely to see such prescribing as a breach of the Dangerous Drugs Regulations 1953 which like the Regulations of 1921 authorized a medical practitioner to possess, supply, etc. controlled drugs 'for the exercise of his practice . . .'. The case involved a London doctor who had issued over 70 prescriptions for heroin for an addict he knew was the patient of another doctor although he had never contacted that doctor to inform him of the fact. Moreover, the first doctor had only seen the addict himself on a dozen or so occasions, being content to hand the prescriptions to the addict's girlfriend, who was herself addicted. In dismissing charges against the doctor, the Magistrate commented (Criminal Law Review 326, 1956):

> It may well be that the patient committed an offence here. It is not for me to decide one way or the other. But to my mind, it would make nonsense of these regulations, which as I see it are designed to give duly qualified medical practitioners absolute discretion as to the way they should treat their patients, and the quantity of drugs that they should prescribe, if I were to hold that these facts amounted to an infringement of the regulations by the defendant. There is nothing in these regulations to which my attention has been directed, which limits the quantity of drugs that may be lawfully prescribed by a doctor.
>
> It may be that this conduct on the part of the defendant was gravely improper; it is not for me to decide any such issue. It may be that this is a matter that might properly be referred to the disciplinary body of the medical profession. . . .

Referring the facts to the General Medical Council was equally unrewarding and produced the reply that while the Council regretted they could not see their way to take any steps against the doctor, they felt strongly the case should be referred to a medical tribunal (provisions for which did not then exist). Although disciplinary action could not therefore be taken against this doctor, market forces in the form of an even more liberal prescriber to whom his regular patients quickly transferred their attention, saw his disappearance from the prescribing scene in 1958. In fairness to the Council it must be remembered that their disciplinary powers were limited to cases of 'serious professional misconduct', or where a doctor had been convicted of a criminal offence, and that in respect of the former the mere act of prescribing drugs liberally did not necessarily amount to 'serious professional misconduct'. This limitation on the Council's powers was explained by Lord Cohen, then President of the General Medical Council in evidence to the Amphetamines Sub-Committee of the Advisory Committee on Drug Dependence in 1969 (Report by the Advisory Committee on Drug Dependence, 1970). He told the Sub-Committee that if a doctor overprescribed drugs because in good faith he regarded this as the right treatment for his patient he would not be guilty of misconduct; or in other words, something done in good faith, even if done wrongly cannot be regarded as 'serious professional misconduct'.

To those closely in touch with the situation the period following the publication of Brain's (1961) comforting picture of opiate dependence in the United Kingdom was one of considerable frustration. The number of new heroin addicts coming to official notice continued to rise at a steady rate and there was sufficient overprescribing by doctors, or under-consumption by addicts, to sustain a flourishing black market in heroin and later cocaine. This black market, consisting of suppliers who were addicts disposing of their own legitimately acquired drugs, posed difficult problems for the police, but while it was supplemented from time to time with the proceeds of thefts from pharmaceutical warehouses, hospitals, doctors' surgeries or retail pharmacies there was no evidence, despite the occasional rumour to the contrary, to suggest that imported illicitly manufactured heroin played any part in the 1958–67 domestic scene. On the contrary, those arrested by the police for the unlawful possession of heroin or cocaine were invariably found in possession of pharmaceutical heroin or cocaine which had come from legitimate sources in the United Kingdom; if illicitly imported heroin had been in circulation in any quantity it is reasonable to expect that the police would have found samples in the possession of at least some addicts.

The continuing deterioration in the situation and the part played in this by the medical profession led to the reconvening of the Interdepartmental Committee in 1963 (Brain, 1965). The Committee's main recommendations, for the restriction of the prescribing of heroin and cocaine to addicts to doctors working at special 'treatment centres' and the notification of addicts to a central authority, are well known and need not be discussed in detail here. What seems to be less well appreciated is that the second Brain Committee was not set up to provide a grand strategy for handling the problem of opiate dependence; that had been the task of its predecessor. The basic purpose of the 1963 enquiry, as is shown by the narrow terms of reference was to provide a solution to the problem of the overprescribing doctor, which the previous enquiry had not identified, let alone resolved. Brain (1965) made no such mistakes, indeed Lord Brain expressed the Committee's task in the simplest terms when, after hearing evidence of one doctor's prescribing practices, he turned to Home Office officials seated at the end of the table and commented: 'Your problem, gentlemen, can be summed up in two words – 'Doctor X'. Nevertheless the Committee's report criticized by implication, if not directly, all those doctors who, 'acting within the law and according to their professional judgment', had provided large amounts of drugs for individual patients. This blanket criticism of those few doctors prepared to enter this very difficult field was grossly unfair, since as Jeffrey (1970) has commented:

> Surprisingly enough however, by 1960, when the major increase in addiction began, the problem was no longer mainly related to the activities of 'script doctors', but rather to those of a few newcomers in the field whose motives were unimpeachable. These were dedicated practitioners, who felt that the young addicts presented a challenge which the rest of the profession was refusing to take up, and who were prepared to put themselves to endless trouble on behalf of the addicts. Inevitably this attitude made them all too ready to give their addicted patients the benefit of the doubt when presented with demand for higher dosage, and the addicts (who are expert manipulators) were quick to take advantage of this. . . . Moreover the fact that only a handful of practitioners was involved meant that as the numbers of addicts increased each began to carry an excessive case-load, and was even less able to devote the necessary time to deciding which were reasonable demands and which were not. . . .

Nevertheless the publicity given to the Committee's Report ensured that in the eyes of the general public these few doctors would be the scapegoats for the increasing heroin addiction problem, even though as has already been pointed out other complex social factors were operating to create the demand for drugs which had not existed from 1920 to 1951. That demand had been growing steadily since 1951, and while the number of known heroin addicts (521) when Brain (1965) reported was small in comparison with the number in some other countries where there was a predominantly illicit heroin black market, the addict population (of known and unknown users) was clearly sufficiently large for the Committee to express their concern at the dilemma, which now faced those responsible for the control of dangerous drugs in the United Kingdom:

> . . . If there is insufficient control it may lead to the spread of addiction – as is happening at present. If, on the other hand, the restrictions are so severe as to prevent or seriously discourage the addict from obtaining supplies from legitimate sources it may lead to the development of an organised traffic. The absence of hitherto such an organised illicit traffic has been attributed largely to the fact that an addict has been able to obtain supplies of drugs legally. . . .

Although Brain (1965) recommended the establishment of treatment centres at which the new generation of heroin and cocaine users would be treated, no detailed blueprint of an ideal centre had been provided, beyond the suggestion that each centre should have facilities for medical treatment, including laboratory investigation and provision for research. It was further suggested that such a centre might form part of a psychiatric hospital or of the psychiatric wing of a general hospital. In the event, after detailed discussions with the medical profession, which were based on estimates that there would be about 1000 addicts seeking treatment in the London area and a further 200 in the rest of the country, arrangements were agreed for the setting up in the London area of fourteen outpatient units, attached in most instances to the major teaching hospitals, and outside London, for provision to be made for addicts to be treated by the normal psychiatric services, except where the number of addicts justified the establishment of a special unit. While most attention had been focused on the situation in London and the Home Counties there were by 1965 small pockets of addiction in some of the major provincial cities. However, these small groups of addicts tended to rely for their supplies on thefts from hospitals and pharmacies, rather than as in London on the generous prescriber. More detailed accounts of the implementation of this aspect of the Brain Committee's recommendations have been provided by Glancy (1972), Leech (1973) and Phillipson (1970).

However, none of these accounts refer to the influence on the planning of the London units of the experience of Dr John Owens and colleagues at All Saints Hospital Birmingham, who after setting up an 'addiction unit' in the autumn of 1964 'offering comprehensive in-patient and out-patient services to people of all ages addicted to, or dependent upon any drug including tobacco', soon found themselves to their surprise dealing with a small but rapidly expanding group of young heroin addicts, the first of whom had arrived from London in the spring of 1965. Throughout the winter of 1965 and spring of 1966 new patients arrived at the Unit at the rate of about twelve a month, many being self-referrals, others being referred by the police or probation service. These comparatively large numbers of very demanding, difficult patients forced the hospital staff to revise their traditional attitudes to the problem and to devise new techniques and approaches. The basic philosophy of the Birmingham approach was to regard treatment 'as a process that would firstly enable the individual to function within the community at a reasonable level', while still using a minimal amount of drugs, prescribed for him or her on a daily basis. It was accepted that it was often unrealistic to expect disturbed youngsters to work and live what was regarded as a normal life, and that if they could live with the aid of social security benefits and keep out of trouble this was a realistic goal and a step in the right direction (Nyman, 1969). By the time the London clinics were ready to open the Birmingham approach had shown promising signs of success and provided useful experience upon which those about to enter the field elsewhere could draw.

WHO TREATS THE ADDICTS – DOCTORS OR CLINICS?

What appeared to some as slow progress in the implementation of Brain's (1965) main recommendation, that only doctors working at treatment centres should in future be permitted to prescribe heroin and cocaine for addicts has been described as 'a remarkable feat of administration and negotiation' (Edwards, 1977). Certainly in the absence of adequate existing facilities to which addicts could be transferred from general practitioners, and in view of the accepted reluctance of most doctors to become involved in what they regarded as a most unrewarding branch of medicine, there was bound to be delay in providing the necessary treatment facilities which had to be capable of accommodating all those heroin addicts who up to then had been treated by general practitioners, as well as an unknown number who, it was hoped, would come forward from the anonymity of the black market. It must also be remembered that with a few exceptions, the only doctors with other than an academic knowledge of the problems involved in treating heroin addiction were the very general practitioners whose involvement the new measures were specifically designed to eliminate. These factors, coupled with the need for legislation meant that the 'new' British approach could not become operative before 16 April 1968. However, some clinics had been treating patients since before that date, having been opened in accordance with the guidance contained in Hospital Memorandum (67) 16 *The Treatment and Supervision of Heroin Addiction* issued on 7 March 1967, which outlined action taken, or proposed, on the recommendations of the second Brain Committee (1965) and described the facilities which hospitals were being asked to provide for persons addicted to heroin. Further guidance followed a year later in Memorandum HM(68) 11 *Dangerous Drugs (Supply to Addicts) Regulations 1968*, which detailed the arrangements for the administration, prescribing and supply of heroin and cocaine to addicts and for dealing with the expected increase in demand for treatment. It is both interesting and important, in the light of present-day practices and the escalating problem, to recall the underlying philosophy which guided the architects of this new approach. One thing was made clear at the outset, and has remained inviolate; the decisions on whether or not to supply an addict with drugs, whether or not to substitute other drugs for those to which he was originally addicted, the assessment of dosage and the method of supply (for example, by prescription, or direct administration), were entirely within the professional discretion and judgement of the doctor in charge of the patient. Treatment policy was not to be dictated by the Ministry of Health, the Home Office or any other government agency, a fact which even now after the innumerable studies of the 'British system' is not fully appreciated even in this country.

However, although there was no centrally imposed treatment policy it is clear that fear of the development of an organized criminal black market was very much in the minds of those planning the new approach. The Brain Committee (1965) had already drawn attention to the dilemma which they saw facing the country (see above); Hospital Memorandum (67) 16 expressed this in slightly different terms which clearly bore the influence of the Birmingham experience, described above:

> Some addicts will not accept withdrawal treatment, at any rate to start with, and complete refusal of supplies will not cure their addiction – it will merely throw them on the black market and encourage the development of an organised illicit traffic on a scale unknown in this country. The aim is to contain the spread of drug addiction by continuing to supply this drug in minimum quantities, where this is necessary in the opinion of the doctor, and where possible to persuade addicts to accept withdrawal treatment.

The rationale of the new approach, which accepted the concept of prescribing heroin for those addicts who did not wish to be withdrawn from the drug, was discussed by Connell (1969), in a paper presented to the Symposium on the Scientific Basis of Drug Dependence in March 1968. In this he expressed the view that a criminally organized heroin supply in the United Kingdom 'must be avoided at all costs', but might well come about if the numbers of addicts were approaching the level at which it would be financially worthwhile for criminal organizations to move in. The point was further emphasized in Hospital Memorandum (68) 11: 'It is most important that hospitals in the National Health Service should deal with all addicts who come to them, so as to reduce the danger of setting up of a new illicit market'.

THE DEVELOPMENT OF HEROIN ADDICTION 1965–68

Yet despite this clear determination that the development of a criminal black market in illicit heroin should be prevented, and the belief that the best means of achieving this was by what has now come to be known 'competitive prescribing', such a black market has now emerged. The first signs of what the future would bring appeared in the period between the publication of the second Brain Committee's report in 1965 and the full implementation of their main recommendations in 1968. This was an important period in a number of respects.

Firstly, it was a period of considerable uncertainty and speculation, particularly within the addict community which was aware of the intention to restrict the prescribing of heroin but had no idea how this was to be implemented and naturally, fearing the worst, began to seek alternative sources of supply. Secondly, there was also during this period a further very large increase in the number of known heroin addicts, which rose from 521 in 1965 to 1299 in 1967. This was due mainly to the arrival of new liberal prescribers to replace some of those who had borne the brunt of addict pressure before 1965, but who had withdrawn from the scene following the publication of the Brain report. Together with those addicts who, for reasons of their own, preferred to remain 'below the surface', these numbers represented a potential market of a size likely, as Connell (1969) suggested, to attract international traffickers, and the first evidence that illicit heroin was available in the United Kingdom in any quantity also came to light in this period.

THE ADVENT OF 'CHINESE' HEROIN

In September 1967, officers of the Metropolitan Police Drugs Squad obtained a small sample of a light brown granular substance which, on analysis, was found to be a mixture of heroin and caffeine. This was part of a consignment from Hong Kong intended for smoking by the Chinese community in London and commonly known as 'No 3' type heroin which was said to retail at £2.50 per grain, or £60–80 per oz wholesale. It was also believed that a small number of London addicts were injecting this impure material intravenously, and positive evidence of this was obtained shortly afterwards when a young addict from Crawley was found in possession of a small quantity. It seems probable that the links between the Chinese heroin smokers and the British mainliners came about by chance and not as a matter of deliberate organization; in fact the names of the British addicts who, it was alleged, had made the initial contact in a billiard hall in Wardour Street were given to the Drugs Branch shortly after 'Chinese' heroin began to appear. It was perhaps not surprising that British addicts, who had been unaccustomed to using heroin in powder form, their supplies having hitherto invariably been of pharmaceutically prepared hypodermic tablets of guaranteed strength and purity, were initially rather suspicious of this new material, but when these suspicions had been overcome the number of persons found in possession of this new form of heroin began to rise. In 1969 just over 60 samples of illicit heroin were submitted to the Metropolitan Police Forensic Science Laboratory, compared with two in 1967 and two in 1968. An additional reason for its growth in popularity was undoubtedly the competitive price; at £1.50 per grain it was cheaper than pharmaceutical heroin which, as a result of the more controlled prescribing by the new treatment centres, was both less readily available and more expensive, at £3 per grain on weekdays and £5–6 at weekends. There were drawbacks, however; the strength and purity of Chinese heroin varied, thus increasing the risk of accidental overdose or infections and samples generally contained less than 50% heroin (the other main ingredient being caffeine). The average contents of a series of samples analysed in 1969, 1970 and 1971 were 38.5%, 42.6%, and 31.6% respectively with the highest at 50% and the lowest at 12%.

This new development not unnaturally attracted considerable attention from the media and focused an unwelcome spotlight on the closely knit Chinese community in the West End of London, which may well have been one of the reasons for the apparent scarcity of illicit heroin in the first few months of 1970. During this period one sample was submitted to the laboratory for analysis. However, by April 1970 Chinese heroin was again circulating on the streets of London's West End, and from that point until the mid-1970s when changes in international trafficking patterns, coupled with concentrated police action against some of the major traffickers resulted in a further retrenchment, it was to remain an established feature of the British opiate black market. The importance of its appearance in this period was that not only did it give British addicts experience of handling material of unknown strength and purity, but it introduced onto the scene, in a larger scale than hitherto, the non-addicted 'pusher'.

METHEDRINE

The third important development, which occurred towards the end of the period between the Brain (1965) report and the introduction of restrictions on prescribing, involved a few of the doctors who had come late onto the prescribing scene. One of these whose authority to prescribe opiates had been withdrawn by the Home Secretary in February 1968, following a conviction for failing to keep records of his purchases of heroin and cocaine, began to prescribe methylamphetamine (in the form of methedrine ampoules), as he was still legally entitled to do. There had been some limited prescribing of this preparation by other doctors prior to this, usually as a substitute for cocaine, but early in 1968 the amount of methedrine circulating in the West End of London increased dramatically. In May 1968, only a month after the new centres had come fully into operation, Drugs Branch inspectors recovered from a number of London pharmacies private prescriptions for a total of 35 248 ampoules. These prescriptions had been issued by eight doctors, one of whom was alone responsible for a total of 24 905 ampoules which he had prescribed for 110 apparently different individuals. The average rate of supply to one of his 'patients' was 46 ampoules per day. As there was still no machinery to deal with the overprescriber *per se*, this abuse could only be curtailed through the willing cooperation of the manufacturers, who, in October 1968, agreed to restrict sales of methylamphetamine ampoules to hospitals. Although this action effectively dealt with the intravenous 'speed' problem the epidemic, as Leech (1973) has pointed out in his entertaining and colourful account of Soho in the late 1960s, had brought together

> the heroin addicts and the wider community of adolescents who were involved with amphetamine use. It was 'Methedrine' use which provided the bridge between the needle culture and the kids in the clubs. It was 'Methedrine' which played the 'escalator' role which is often, wrongly, attributed to cannabis. It was 'Methedrine' which made the process of 'fixing' an integral part of the West End drug culture. The West End was not the same after 'Methedrine'; it was more destructive, more hopeless, more needle centred.

OVERPRESCRIBING IN THE CLINICS

One of the first priorities of the new generation of prescribers was to reduce the amount of legitimate heroin and cocaine available for sale in the black market and in the case of cocaine, which produced little physical dependence, this was achieved rapidly. However, heroin presented different and more difficult problems, and there is little doubt that in the early days there was considerable overprescribing by clinics, although not on the spectacular scale of the pre-Brain (1965) era. That there was overprescribing by the clinics was hardly surprising, given that there was no simple foolproof scientific method for assessing an addict's drug requirements and that in this early period, in the clinics' history, the addicts' experience of dealing with doctors usually far outweighed that of the doctors in 'treating' them. The most telling evidence that the clinics had a marked effect on the black market was the gradual increase in the price of pharmaceutically produced hypodermic tablets of heroin, which for years had been stable at six tablets (each of

10 mg) for £1. As already mentioned, by the spring of 1968 the weekday price of legitimate heroin had trebled, and within a short time prices of £1 for one tablet were being quoted. The present-day scarcity of pharmaceutical heroin is reflected in the price of £6–7 for one ampoule of freeze-dried material.

METHADONE AS A HEROIN SUBSTITUTE

Apart from the general reduction in the size of individual doses prescribed to addicts, the main change in the prescribing pattern introduced by the clinics post-April 1968 was the use of methadone as a substitute for heroin. Although the work of Dole and Nyswander was well known in the United Kingdom there had been little use of methadone here in the treatment of addiction. It had, in fact, been proposed initially that only methadone would be prescribed by the clinics, but this plan was abandoned in the light of Home Office fears that such an inflexible approach would discourage addicts from attending the clinics and would in all probability accelerate the development of a criminal black market. Nevertheless there was a gradual move by most clinics towards methadone substitution, using the drug in injectable rather than the oral form favoured in the United States. Methadone was, and still is, unpopular with experienced addicts, who, although finding the injection solution a useful preparation for flushing out their syringes, initially exchanged their ampoules for other drugs or sold them in the market; the proceeds from these were then used to buy illicit heroin. The customers for these unwanted ampoules were often young persons coming onto the fringe of the addict scene, and by 1970 there was a significant number of primary methadone addicts approaching the clinics. This naturally alarmed the clinics, but their proposal that general practitioners should be advised against prescribing methadone by injection for addicts had to be dropped when a survey by the Home Office of methadone prescribing in the London area demonstrated beyond doubt that the major sources of the surplus were the clinics themselves and not general practitioners. The extent to which clinics have substituted methadone for heroin is strikingly illustrated in Figure 3.1 which also shows how injectable methadone has been replaced by oral forms of the drug. In the early days most clinics had their own individual oral methadone formulation, but following discussions at the periodic conferences of clinic consultants which were instituted by the Ministry of Health a standard formulation was agreed.

INCREASING INTRAVENOUS USE OF BARBITURATES

At about the same time as the wave of new methadone addicts began to emerge in 1969 there were disturbing signs of increasing intravenous use of barbiturates usually in the form of Tuinal or Nembutal. Abuse of these drugs had, up to then, been mainly by persons of middle age, although barbiturates had been a common addition to prescriptions for

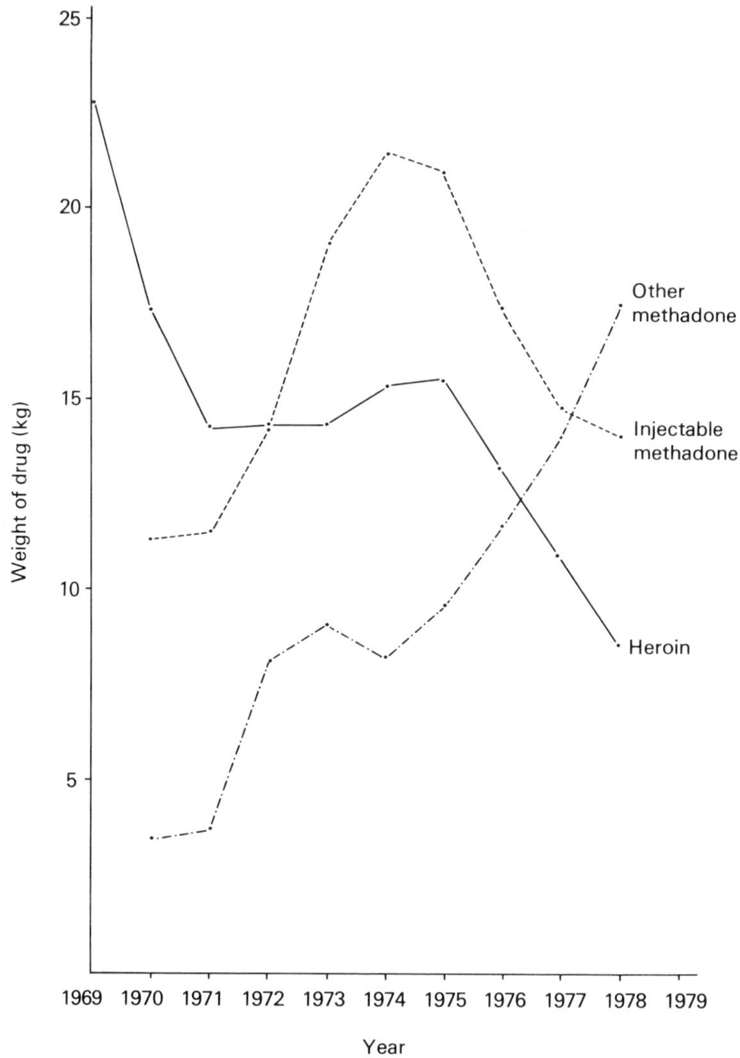

Figure 3.1 Drugs prescribed by outpatient clinics in England and Wales

heroin issued to addicts but for oral rather than intravenous use. The new post-1968 abusers were often heroin addicts supplementing their prescribed quantities of heroin or methadone with barbiturates, obtained from doctors on a casual or regular basis, by thefts from retail pharmacies, or by forged prescriptions. In addition to the normal serious hazards of physical and psychological dependence and withdrawal associated with barbiturate use, the intravenous injection of material intended for administration orally brought an increased incidence of abcesses, infections and ulcers and, as Leech (1973) has pointed out, a physical and mental deterioration of the West End street addict which was a source of concern to all the agencies working in the area. This concern was eventually voiced in the House of Commons during the Second Reading on the Misuse of Drugs Bill in March 1970 as a result of which the Home Secretary referred the question of whether or not barbiturates should be controlled under the Bill to the Advisory Committee on Drug Dependence. The Committee found that the problem of intravenous injection of barbiturates was mainly confined to London and the Home Counties, although there was evidence from the police that small groups of addicts existed in some other parts of the country. A survey conducted by the Department of Health and Social Security of drug treatment centres and their associated casualty units identified 284 barbiturate needle-users during a 3-month period, while the Association for the Prevention of Addiction's Day Centre in the West End was, during 1969, seeing an average of 40–50 addicts per day, many of whom were injecting barbiturates. The Advisory Committee were unable to identify any special reason for the sudden emergence of this group nor could they establish that 'unduly severe restrictions on the prescribing of heroin or methadone to narcotic addicts was a significant factor' in the outbreak. They did, however, recommend that barbiturates should be subject to a measure of control under the proposed new legislation, but in the event time did not allow for the necessary consultation with the professional bodies and the Misuse of Drugs Act 1971 came into effect with barbiturates excluded from its provisions.

CAMPAIGN ON THE USE AND RESTRICTION OF BARBITURATES (CURB)

Further consideration of the barbiturate problem became one of the first tasks of the Advisory Council on the Misuse of Drugs, appointed under the 1971 Act and this led to the setting up of the Campaign on the Use and Restriction of Barbiturates (CURB) in September 1975. The primary purpose of this 2-year campaign was to reduce the availability of barbiturate preparations to misusers, by persuading doctors to curtail their prescribing of these preparations and to warn members of the public of the dangers of depending on them for inducing sleep. However, by 1978 the Advisory Council felt satisfied that a serious problem of barbiturate misuse by young people continued to exist, and that there might now be a favourable climate of opinion, particularly within the medical profession, for the acceptance of control of barbiturate preparations under the 1971 Act. Detailed consideration of how this was best achieved has therefore been resumed.

DICONAL ABUSE

The growing abuse of illicit heroin, methadone and barbiturates, described above, was first detected in London and the Home Counties, spreading later in varying degree to the provinces. In the case of Diconal abuse this trend was reversed with the first indication that this was a preparation with considerable addict appeal coming from the North of England. Dipipanone, its active ingredient, had been placed under control in 1954 and had been available in the United Kingdom in the form of a 25 mg injection and an oral tablet also containing 25 mg of the drug and 50 mg cyclizine. The latter was withdrawn in 1961 in favour of Diconal which contained only 10 mg dipipanone and 30 mg cyclizine. Throughout the period from 1954 only a limited amount of therapeutic abuse of dipipanone had come to the notice of the Home Office, but in 1970 a small number of notifications of addiction were received from a treatment centre in the North of England. Enquiries revealed that although there had been some abuse of Diconal in the area these notifications were in fact of patients who were being given the drug after a number of other oral preparations had been tried, as a means of weaning them off opiates. Although Diconal was intended to be taken orally the local drug squad soon reported that the addicts preferred to crush and inject the tablets, thereby producing a 'buzz' or 'high' which was heroin-like, though of shorter duration, and also risking the physical complications associated with the intravenous injection of an oral preparation.

In the summer of 1971 an outbreak of Diconal abuse came to notice on the south coast of England, but as far as could be determined there was no connection between this group of addicts and the northern group. The south coast addicts were largely supplied on the prescriptions of one general practitioner who appeared willing to prescribe Diconal regularly for any young person, whether on his NHS list or not, who complained of backache or dysmenorrhea. These supplies were supplemented with Diconal obtained by forged prescriptions or stolen from legitimate stocks. The 'retirement' of this doctor from the prescribing scene, following police and Home Office intervention, resulted in the addicts pestering other general practitioners in the area, from many of whom they were able to obtain temporary resident prescriptions for small quantities. In December 1971 a further outbreak occurred in another south coast town and was similarly fuelled by the prescriptions of an elderly general practitioner. Some of his patients came from as far away as London, and some were also concurrently receiving methadone from the local treatment centre, but as far as he was concerned there was a valid medical reason, usually backache, for each prescription. Following the successful prosecution of some of these patients this doctor also ceased to prescribe Diconal.

Within a comparatively short space of time Diconal abuse had spread to most areas of the country where there were injecting addicts and today this preparation continues to be a major factor in the British opiate abuse scene. Although it was not known at the time the Republic of Ireland was in 1970 also experiencing a problem with Diconal abuse (Kelly, 1972); the sources of supply in both countries were the same, but whereas in the United Kingdom legitimate prescriptions from doctors provided addicts with their first experience of this drug, the Irish addicts had initially obtained their supplies by theft from retail pharmacies, turning to medical prescriptions in 1971. The effect of medical involvement was to accelerate the growth of the problem which by November 1971 had reached such proportions that the marketing of the preparation was temporarily suspended, except for supplies to a few hospitals caring for terminal patients. Apart from the United Kingdom and the Republic of Ireland the only other country to encounter this problem appears to be South Africa, where in early 1981 there were press reports of overdose deaths, from the administration of Wellconal (the name under which Diconal is marketed abroad).

The abuse of Diconal is of interest in two other respects. Firstly, its appearance in the UK illicit market occurred, as has been seen above, at a very important time. The hitherto almost exclusively heroin and cocaine scene was changing into one in which addicts were regularly using a variety of drugs including illicit heroin, methadone and barbiturates, following the reduction in the 'grey' market of pharmaceutical heroin, as a result of the more responsible prescribing by the treatment centres since April 1968. In such circumstances, the discovery of a substitute for heroin, albeit an inferior one, which could be obtained from doctors with little difficulty, rapidly became common knowledge throughout the addict community, and the increasing popularity of this preparation with abusers began to be reflected in the official statistics (Table 3.1). It is also interesting to speculate that the emergence of Diconal at this particular time may have provided a buffer which delayed the growth of the illicit heroin market which was to come later and which was already beginning to affect some other countries in western Europe.

Table 3.1 *Diconal (dipipanone)*

	1970	*1971*	*1972*	*1973*	*1974*	*1975*	*1976*	*1977*	*1978*	*1979*	*1980*
Number of addicts receiving dipipanone at 31 December	45	49	37	48	75	132	158	241	310	381	399
Number of first notifications for dipipanone	not available				52	125	130	232	273	320	349
Number of persons convicted of dipipanone offences	not available			198	369	409	361	378	498	453	449

DICONAL AND THE DOCTOR

The second aspect of the Diconal problem which is of importance is that it refocused attention on the role of the doctor as a source of supply to the black market. Although thefts from pharmacies and forged prescriptions contributed to the availability of Diconal, the principal source, as with heroin in the 1960s, was medical prescriptions. However, unlike the period before Brain (1965), when the problem had been of a very few doctors prescribing generous quantities of heroin and cocaine, the Diconal problem involved a much larger number of doctors in various parts of the country who, with a few exceptions, did not prescribe spectacularly large quantities for individuals. In most instances, their involvement stemmed from their failure to associate Diconal with addiction, as they would have done if asked for morphine or heroin; some even failed to do so after checking the latest edition of MIMS, which clearly showed that Diconal was 'a controlled drug', and their suspicions usually only began to be roused when they realized they had suddenly acquired a sizeable group of young 'temporary residents' suffering from backache or some similar conditions. (In one instance an elderly doctor in West London acquired over 70 Diconal patients within the space of a fortnight, and another doctor in a period of 2½ months prescribed *with no enquiry* just over 11 000 Diconal tablets, 2000 Ritalin (methylphenidate) tablets and 1300 ampoules/tablets of methadone to some 200 individuals.) Neither did these doctors realize that the tablets they prescribed had a considerable black market value (in 1980 about £5–6 per tablet in London) and would probably be injected. In fairness to these doctors, whose motives for prescribing were in most cases beyond reproach, it must be said that addicts demonstrated an uncanny ability to single out the more vulnerable members of the profession, often the elderly single-handed practitioner with little or no experience of the modern non-therapeutic addict, and who at a later stage in the relationship could be pressurized by the addict to continue prescribing, even though by then he might well realize he was being manipulated.

As in the pre-Brain (1965) period there was no machinery, in the early days of the Diconal problem, to deal satisfactorily with prescribing where the prescribers' motives were suspect, let alone where the prescribing was well-intentioned but naive. The Dangerous Drugs Act 1967 had provided for the re-establishment of tribunal machinery but this was to police the restrictions on the prescribing of heroin and cocaine to addicts and not the general prescribing of controlled drugs. (Brain (1965) had recommended that breaches of the regulations limiting the prescribing of heroin and cocaine should be the responsibility of the General Medical Council but the Council were reluctant to accept this, even if appropriately empowered to do so and favoured instead the establishment of a body composed largely, if not wholly, of persons with special expertise in the field of drug dependence.) This meant that the only way of tackling the naive prescriber of Diconal was to draw his attention to the consequences of his prescribing, that he was undoubtedly, if unwittingly, contributing to the black market, in the hope that he would withdraw from the scene. Unfortunately as soon as one prescriber was successfully persuaded to stop, or exercise greater control over his prescribing, addicts would discover another sympathetic and willing practitioner and the process would have to be repeated.

THE AMPHETAMINES SUB-COMMITTEE OF THE ADVISORY COMMITTEE ON DRUG DEPENDENCE

The situation was, however, eased by the provision in the Misuse of Drugs Act 1971 of machinery whereby action could be taken against any practitioner who prescribed or supplied controlled drugs 'in an irresponsible manner'. If there were sufficient grounds for believing that a practitioner was prescribing in such a manner the Secretary of State was empowered to refer the facts to a special tribunal which, if satisfied that the practitioner had been so acting, could recommend that a direction be made against him prohibiting from prescribing, supplying such drugs as were specified in the direction. The restoration of the safeguard, which nearly 50 years previously the Rolleston Committee had felt it necessary to recommend, was largely the result of the work of the Amphetamines Sub-Committee of the Advisory Committee on Drug Dependence. This Sub-Committee had been appointed just as the methylamphetamine epidemic, described above, was being brought to an end, 'to examine the medical, social and legal aspects of the use and misuse of amphetamines and similar central nervous system stimulant drugs'. They were therefore very much aware that the doctor's prescription pad could be a major source of some drugs of abuse. Like the Brain Committee in 1965, the Sub-Committee felt it would be desirable to extend the powers of the General Medical Council, as the body concerned with professional standards, to enable the Council to deal with reckless overprescribing, but that if this was not acceptable special tribunals should be set up, as recommended in the Rolleston report. In the event, despite pressure exerted on the General Medical Council in Parliament and elsewhere, the Council adhered to its already stated view that it would be better to establish specialist tribunals to deal with allegations of improper prescribing. Provision was therefore made in the Misuse of Drugs Act 1971 for the restoration of the tribunals and, additionally, for a special emergency procedure, also recommended by the Sub-Committee on Amphetamines, whereby in particularly serious cases where there had been reckless overprescribing, liable to create a public health problem, the Secretary of State, on the advice of a small panel of suitably qualified doctors, could temporarily suspend a doctor's authority to prescribe controlled drugs, pending reference of the facts to a full tribunal. It will be remembered that the first Brain Committee (1961) were impressed by the difficulties of establishing special tribunals to deal with overprescribing and advised against their restoration; to date the Misuse of Drugs Act machinery has been used on nine occasions (mainly for Diconal and stimulants such as Ritalin) with the emergency provisions being used twice, and none of the difficulties foreseen by Brain (1961) have been encountered in practice. It must also be noted that over the past 12 years the General Medical Council Disciplinary Committee have erased or suspended from the Medical Register the names of a number of practitioners who have prescribed controlled drugs otherwise than in the course of *bona fide* treatment, such as to constitute in the view of the Committee 'serious professional misconduct'.

RITALIN AND COCAINE

Methylphenidate (Ritalin) and cocaine are two drugs pharmacologically outside the terms of reference of this review, but nevertheless because of their use by opiate abusers cannot be excluded entirely. Ritalin, in particular, is frequently used in conjunction with Diconal to prolong the 'high' of the latter, and like Diconal is easily obtained from doctors to treat depression usually brought on by some personal tragedy such as the loss of a close relative in a road accident. For example, an illustration of the ease with which Ritalin can be obtained from unsuspecting practitioners was provided in 1979 by a young woman who, with a male associate, each using a variety of names, and background stories, were able in a 5-month period to obtain prescriptions totalling over 10 000 tablets of Ritalin from about 100 doctors in the Harley Street area of London. The couple disposed of the tablets through 'runners' who sold them in the West End of London.

There have been three periods when cocaine abuse in the United Kingdom has reached significant proportions. The first of these was during and after the First World War when it became a popular drug in London society. The death of a young actress in November 1918 after the Victory Ball aroused considerable public interest in the extent and nature of drug abuse in those circles, but abuse of and traffic in cocaine soon declined and by 1927 the annual number of prosecutions for offences involving cocaine had dropped to two. The second 'outbreak' of cocaine abuse occurred in the late 1950s when it was introduced to the growing circle of heroin addicts by a doctor who felt it would provide sufficient stimulation to enable these addicts to work, or to restore the 'buzz' or 'high' which many of the recently arrived heroin addicts from Canada claimed they did not experience with pharmaceutically pure heroin. In return for this bonus the addicts were expected to make serious efforts to decrease their intake of heroin, but few of them did, and as can be seen from the addict statistics for the period (Table 3.2) the number of persons taking both heroin and cocaine rose dramatically. The implementation in April 1968 of the Brain (1965) recommendation to limit the prescribing of heroin and cocaine to addicts to doctors at treatment centres effectively dealt with this problem. The treatment-centre doctors rapidly discontinued the prescribing of cocaine, reducing the number of notified users of cocaine (alone or in combination with other drugs) from 564 in 1968 to 81 who were receiving this drug in the course of treatment on 31 December 1969.

But as cocaine use amongst addicts dwindled, its use amongst the 'jet set' (the 1970s equivalent of the cocaine users of the 1920s) increased, and it was soon obvious that this was part of a worldwide revival of interest in this drug. Unlike the previous period, when cocaine was prescribed by doctors, the new generation of abusers relied entirely on illicit supplies originating in South America and smuggled into the country by a variety of routes and ruses. Moreover, unlike the addicts of the 1960s the new users sniffed (or 'snorted') the drug often through rolled up banknotes, a method which after some time can lead to the erosion of the nasal septum. Statistics of prosecutions and seizures (see Table 3.3) provide some indication of the increasing use and demand for cocaine but perhaps the most telling evidence of its widespread popularity was that provided by a London doctor recently who asked if he was required to notify all the cocaine addicts he met socially! Cocaine abuse is also growing in western Europe, parts of the Middle East and North America where its use is escalating particularly amongst the 18–25 age group, a trend which is reflected in the US authorities' estimate that in 1979 cocaine displaced cannabis as the principal producer of illicit drug income in that country (United Nations, 1980).

Table 3.2 *Addict statistics (1957–69)*

	1957	*1958*	*1959*	*1960*	*1961*	*1962*	*1963*	*1964*	*1965*	*1966*	*1967*	*1968*	*1969*
Total number of addicts in the year	359	442	454	437	470	532	635	753	927	1349	1729	2782	2881
Number of addicts taking heroin*	66	62	68	94	132	175	237	342	521	899	1299	2240	1417
Number of addicts taking cocaine*	16	25	30	52	84	112	171	211	311	443	462	564	81†

*alone or in combination with other drugs, the most frequent combination being heroin and cocaine
† receiving cocaine at 31 December 1969

Table 3.3 *Cocaine seizures/offences*

	1970	*1971*	*1972*	*1973*	*1974*	*1975*	*1976*	*1977*	*1978*	*1979*	*1980*
Total quantity of cocaine seized in kg	0.2	0.3	0.6	6.4	10.4	7.1	9.9	13.7	16.1	24.0	40.2
Number of persons convicted of cocaine offences	122	119	193	181	375	379	327	309	348	331	476

CHANGES IN THE PATTERN OF OPIATE ABUSE

It is clear from the above account that there have been substantial changes in the pattern of opiate abuse in the United Kingdom since the second Brain Committee (1965) sat. Changes in patterns of abuse are not necessarily accompanied by an increase in the extent of abuse, but in the light of what has happened since 1965, is the widely held view that the British opiate problem has been quantitatively contained really justified? The accurate measurement of what is essentially an illicit activity presents considerable problems, but there are a number of indicators which despite their individual limitations provide a reliable picture of what is happening.

The first of these is the information provided by the notifications of addicts submitted by doctors to the Chief Medical Officer at the Home Office in accordance with regulations first introduced in February 1968. The statutory notification of addiction, the primary object of which was seen as the need to detect readily those addicts obtaining drugs concurrently from two doctors, had been rejected by the Rolleston Committee on the grounds that the size of the problem at the time did not warrant such a measure, that it would 'impair the confidential character of the relationship of doctor and patient', that the Home Office while accepting that notification would be useful did not feel it was essential for detecting persons obtaining 'dual supplies' and, rather naively, that the recently introduced restrictions on supply and greater care by practitioners in the use of drugs in treatment, would 'go a long way to extinguish the evil'.

The first Brain Committee (1961) did not address themselves to the question of notification but firmly rejected the idea of 'registration' which they felt had 'been taken in error to mean that addicts in Great Britain are entitled to receive supplies of dangerous drugs on prescription and that this involves the registration of the addict with some central authority'. However, the second Brain Committee (1965), drawing an analogy between addiction and infectious disease, proposed that there should be compulsory confidential notification of addiction to a central authority, although they, like their predecessors, rejected the concept of registration which 'might seem to imply that the addict is officially recognised as having the right to an approved quantity of dangerous drugs'. The purpose of notification, as Brain (1965) saw it, was to provide medical practitioners with a ready reference point to check whether a particular addict had already been notified and to obtain further particulars about an addict's history. This remains the primary purpose of the notification procedure as currently practised, but clearly the information provided by doctors about the numbers and types of addicts seeking treatment has an additional intelligence and statistical value. At present the Regulations require that any doctor seeking a person he considers, or has reasonable grounds to suspect, is addicted, and regardless of whether or not he prescribes, to furnish in writing to the Chief Medical Officer at the Home Office, within 7 days of the attendance, the name, address, sex, date of birth, and NHS number of that person, the date of the attendance and the name of the drug involved. The information about notification is treated in confidence and is of course, safeguarded by the Official Secrets Act. Notification has no legal consequences for the addict and as mentioned above is not to be equated with 'registration'; the treatment an addict receives from his doctor remains entirely a matter for that doctor, regardless of whether or not the addict has been notified and is subject only to the limitations on the prescribing of heroin and cocaine mentioned earlier.

NOTIFICATION

The main limitations of statistics based on notifications are that even 13 years after the notification became a statutory requirement not all doctors are aware of their obligations. There is confusion about the circumstances under which notification is required; for example, some doctors believe they must notify only if they prescribe, others are uncertain about the implications for their patient of notification, and shelter behind a diagnosis of 'personality disorder' rather than addiction, or a conclusion that the patient's drug involvement does not meet the criteria of addiction laid down in the Regulations. But accepting these limitations, there is clear evidence (see Table 3.4) of a steady increase in the number of addicts coming to notice annually, and that this increase has accelerated since 1977. From 1970 until 1977 the average annual increases in the total number of addicts coming to notice throughout the year was 4.4%, whereas the 1978 total showed an increase of 14.2% in the previous year, and the 1979 total an increase of 16.5% on 1978.

Table 3.4 *Notified addicts*

	1970	*1971*	*1972*	*1973*	*1974*	*1975*	*1976*	*1977*	*1978*	*1979*	*1980*
Total number of addicts known during year*	2657	2762	2936	3023	3252	3425	3474	3605	4116	4787	5107
Number of new cases notified during year	711	774	800	807	870	922	984	1109	1347	1597	1600
Number of former addicts renotified during year	484	562	587	599	566	536	541	622	753	778	841

*This figure corresponds to the 'total addicts' figure in statistics for years 1958–68, i.e. before the practice began of showing total under treatment on 31 December

Analysis of the notifications shows several other interesting trends. Firstly, whereas of the first notifications (that is, of persons not previously known to the Home Office) submitted in 1970 only some 46% claimed addiction to heroin and 33% addiction to methadone, at the time of approaching a doctor, by 1980 these proportions had changed to 72.1% and 9.6% respectively; since comparatively little heroin is now being prescribed by the treatment centres, this can only mean the presence of a substantial black market in this drug. In 1971 and 1972 when there was considerable concern about the alleged ease with which addicts were said to be able to buy 'Chinese' heroin, there was a similar rise in the heroin first notifications, with just over two-thirds of the new addicts claiming to be using heroin; in 1972, however, when, for reasons already indicated above, there was believed to be less Chinese heroin available on the street only half the new notifications were in respect of heroin. This shows that the notification procedure can be of value in supporting intelligence from the street, which often tends to be discounted because it is impressionistic.

The first notifications also show that after a gradual decline since 1970 in the number of addicts under the age of 20 being notified, this trend has been reversed and this is also supported by street evidence which suggests that the young have once more found heroin to be an attractive drug, although there are grounds for believing that addicts in this age-group are more reluctant than others tò place themselves in situations where they have to be 'notified'. This is particularly true in respect of the increasing use of heroin and cocaine amongst young persons from the higher social classes, who not surprisingly are reluctant for their names to become known to the authorities. This trend towards a younger addict population may appear to be in contrast to the statement in the Home Office Statistical Bulletin for 1979 that the figures showed a continuation of the gradual increase in the average age of notified addicts. The increasing average age, on which that statement is based, is that of addicts known to be receiving drugs on 31 December of each year. Since this relates to addicts in treatment and, as some have been in treatment since the clinics opened, it is not surprising that the average age of this population should be increasing.

Another interesting trend, revealed by a close examination of the first notifications is that in 1979 for the first time more addicts were notified by general practitioners (including police surgeons) than by treatment centres and hospitals (44.8% against 38.2%). In 1970 just over 45% of first notifications came from treatment centres or hospitals and only 14.6% from general practitioners. To some extent this increase is the result of various campaigns which have been undertaken to make general practitioners aware of their legal responsibilities but there is nevertheless good supportive evidence from other sources that more general practitioners, including those in the private sector, are becoming involved in the problems of the drug addict.

TREATMENT CENTRES

That addicts should now be exerting more pressure on general practitioners is not altogether surprising. In 1968 when treatment centres officially came into existence the opiate problem was confined almost entirely to London and the Home Counties, and except in Birmingham and a few other provincial areas where special centres on the London model were established, arrangements were made for the few addicts expected to surface to be treated by the ordinary hospital psychiatric services. The main consequence of this was that whereas in London and the other special treatment areas addicts could reasonably expect initially to receive prescriptions for heroin or methadone in one form or another, an addict approaching the designated addiction treatment facilities in a provincial area had no such expectations. Treatment approaches varied from a willingness to prescribe heroin or methadone, or more recently Diconal, to the more usual offer of immediate inpatient withdrawal treatment, or (albeit less frequently), a blank refusal to prescribe any medicament other than minor tranquillizers. Nor is it entirely unknown for a general practitioner to be advised by the local consultant that his patient should 'get on a train and go back to London'. Certainly prescribing even on a temporary basis was not the general order of the day in the provinces, and as addicts began to appear in these areas throughout the 1970s many, faced with the lack of treatment acceptable to them, sought supplies of drugs, often Diconal, from local general practitioners, by breaking into retail pharmacies or doctors' surgeries, by forged prescriptions or by pooling their finances and sending one of their group to London to obtain supplies.

By the late 1970s the London treatment centres had amongst themselves agreed two major changes in policy which were also inevitably to increase the pressure on general practitioners. The first of these was the decision not to prescribe injectable drugs, either heroin or methadone, to either new patients or to former patients returning from prison or a period of abstinence; instead patients would be offered oral methadone. The other was the decision of the London treatment centres to accept patients only from a rigid catchment area, which meant that new addicts from the Home Counties would in future have to rely on local, and often 'non-prescribing', facilities. The undoubted effect of these has been to encourage the reappearance of the private practitioner, prepared to prescribe injectable drugs to new patients.

It has been argued that the decision to stop prescribing injectables has been a major factor in the rapid development since 1977 of a criminally organized black market in heroin, but just as it would be wrong to blame the explosion of heroin abuse in the 1960s entirely on the prescribers of that period, so it would be wrong to blame the present increase in heroin abuse entirely on the changed prescribing policies of the London clinics. That there is a relationship between prescribing and the black market is undeniable; too generous a supply changes an addict's status on the market from customer to supplier, whereas a policy of no prescribing or of prescribing drugs which the addict does not want, merely encourages him to seek supplies elsewhere. It was the misfortune of the London clinics that these decisions were taken at the same time as there were some subtle, and some not so subtle, changes taking place in the international trafficking patterns.

HEROIN SOURCES

SOUTH-EAST ASIA

Although as already mentioned, South-east Asian heroin had become a regular feature of the London black market, by 1969 there were very few reports of this substance appearing elsewhere in western Europe. One reason for this was that there was a sufficiently large local market, which included the US troops in Vietnam, to absorb most of the increased production from the notorious 'Golden Triangle'. Production in that area had been expanded to compensate for the ban on the cultivation of the opium poppy in Turkey in 1971, which had effectively removed, at least for a time, one of the major sources of morphine base for the clandestine laboratories in France which supplied heroin to North America. With the end of the Vietnam war far eastern traffickers began to look for new markets, and as North America was then being supplied largely from Mexico and South America, quickly realized the potential of western Europe. Moreover the Chinese communities in some of these countries, but particularly in the Netherlands where additionally penalties for drug offences were lower than elsewhere in Europe, provided a ready-made cohesive and virtually impenetrable trafficking network. In 1975 reports reaching Interpol Headquarters in Paris showed that nearly 300 kg of South-east Asian heroin had been seized in western Europe, a total which was to double in 1976, when the seizure of over 630 kg was reported to Interpol; in their Annual Report for 1976 the International Narcotics Control Board commented on the very serious increase in the misuse of heroin in the Federal Republic of Germany and to a lesser, but nevertheless significant extent, in Belgium, France, Italy, the Netherlands, Sweden and Switzerland. By this time also Amsterdam had acquired the unenviable reputation of being the 'drug capital of Europe', with heroin reaching the city from Thailand and Malaysia by complex routes which frequently involved the United Kingdom as a transit point. However, by 1976 following seizures of No 3-type heroin by the Metropolitan Police Drugs Squad it was evident that this country was no longer solely a transit point and that there was a steady importation of illicit heroin, not only direct from the Far East but also from Amsterdam, to which some enterprising British addicts travelled for supplies.

MIDDLE EAST

Following successful police operations in London which resulted in lengthy prison sentences for some Chinese traffickers, and a shortfall in the production of opium in the 'Golden Triangle' as a result of two successive years of drought, South-east Asian heroin became less readily available in the British markets. However, towards the end of 1976 there were indications of heroin abuse amongst Iranian students in the United Kingdom, and as was perhaps to be expected within a short while British addicts were using heroin from this new source. The internal troubles in Iran, which led to a breakdown in law and order, undoubtedly contributed to the increased flow of heroin from that area, some of which was used by Iranians leaving the country, as a means of transferring their financial assets, but although since the middle of 1980 there has been a drastic reduction in the amount of heroin entering the United Kingdom from Iran, other areas of the Middle East have more than compensated for this reduction. It is in fact one of the major items of concern for the international, as well as national, control agencies that the Middle East has in recent years become an important source of illicitly produced heroin which is being imported into western Europe and North America in increasing quantities. To date three different types of qualities of Middle East heroin have been encountered in the United Kingdom, a brown lumpy powder containing between 50 and 90% heroin, a fine cream powder containing between 40 and 70% heroin, and very variable beige-to-light-brown material, appearing as powders, granules or earthy agglomerates containing only 20–30% heroin.

Table 3.5 *Heroin seizures/offences*

	1970	*1971*	*1972*	*1973*	*1974*	*1975*	*1976*	*1977*	*1978*	*1979*	*1980*
Total quantity of heroin seized in kg	1.6	1.1	13.1	3.3	2.8	6.9	20.2	26.6	60.8	44.9	38.2
Number of persons convicted of heroin offences	232	520	532	435	444	393	464	393	483	520	751
Number of first notifications	not available				531	527	606	614	859	1117	1151

EFFECTS ON THE UNITED KINGDOM OF INTERNATIONAL CHANGES

Apart from the increased abuse of heroin, already mentioned, the extent to which the United Kingdom has been affected by these international changes is seen from the seizures of heroin made by HM Customs and Excise (Table 3.5). Until 1979 there were clear indications that most of the heroin seized at the ports was intended for re-export to other western European countries or North America, but in 1979 there was evidence that of the total quantity seized about 70% was intended for domestic consumption in the United Kingdom. Most of this was of Near or Middle Eastern origin unlike previous years when the majority of heroin seized originated in the Far East. This clearly demonstrates that the United Kingdom is now seen as a market for illicit heroin from this source and raises the inevitable speculation about the quantity which must be successfully evading import controls each year. The stable price of illicit heroin, which is in itself a good indication of availability, and the general comments from the street about how easy it is currently to obtain the drug, suggests that despite the very considerable successes of HM Customs and Excise enough heroin is reaching the addict community to satisfy current demands and that any increases in that demand can be accommodated quite easily.

It is not surprising that the situation described above, of a steadily growing addict population, increasingly fed by illicit supplies derived from international rather than domestic sources, should prompt questions about the present-day relevance of the traditional British approach to the treatment of opiate addiction, with its emphasis on prescribing as an integral part of that approach. The aim of the Brain (1965) proposals was to prevent the development of such an international type black market, while at the same time offering the addicts adequate opportunities for treatment. As Jeffery (1970), writing shortly after the Regulations had been made giving effect to the Brain proposals, explained:

> It is clear, however, that a major factor (in stemming the growth of drug abuse) will be the degree of success achieved by the doctors in the treatment centres in assessing the minimum dosage needed by those addicts attending the centres who are not prepared to undergo withdrawal immediately, and for whom heroin continues to be prescribed. The hope is, of course, that if that minimum dosage can be assessed accurately the surplus heroin at present available for supply to others will be eliminated, so that no new cases of addiction will develop, while those addicts at present dependent on the surplus will themselves turn to the treatment centres. That hope, however, will be frustrated if accurate assessment proves impossible; overprescribing would result in a continuation of the existing situation (although doubtless on a reduced scale) while under-prescribing could drive the addicts already attending the treatment centres to seek illicit supplementary supplies, and discourage those addicts not yet attending centres from doing so – with the almost certain result that the international traffickers would find it worth their while to extend their activities to this country.

CONCLUSIONS

That the present situation is not what the architects of the treatment-centre scheme hoped to achieve is undeniable; whether it is a direct consequence of the measures introduced in 1968 is debatable. There are those who would agree that the Brain (1965) philosophy, resting 'on a daringly simple reading of how a highly complex system would respond to certain influences' (Edwards, 1977) was doomed to failure; others would argue that the Brain philosophy was never given a fair trial because from the outset there has been a steady move by the treatment centres away from the prescribing of heroin and more recently of all injectable drugs (see Table 3.1), with the result that faced with the prospect of a diminishing supply of the drug of their choice from traditional prescription sources, addicts have come increasingly to rely on a black market which places no demands on them beyond an ability to pay for their drugs. Once established, as the experience of other countries clearly shows, such a market, motivated largely by commercial considerations, will be almost impossible to eliminate, and it will be the ability of that market to maintain a reliable supply of good quality, reasonably priced heroin which will now determine the future pattern of opiate abuse in this country, rather than the prescribing policies of the clinics. At best 'competitive prescribing' can only hope to attract addicts away from the black market at a faster rate than they are being recruited. The emergence of a criminal black market adds a new and sinister dimension to the opiate abuse in this country, and will move the problem away from the medical area where it has been for the past 60 years into the areas of enforcement and, in the long term, prevention. The heroin problem of the 1960s was seen as 'a challenge to the practice of medicine' (Connell, 1969); the problem of the 1980s is very much a challenge to the whole community.

REFERENCES

Bean, P. (1974). *The Social Control of Drugs*, (Oxford: Martin Robertson)
Brain Committee (1961). *Drug Addiction, Report of the Interdepartmental Committee.* (London: HMSO)
Brain Committee (1965). *Drug Addiction: The Second Report of the Interdepartmental Committee.* (London: HMSO)
Connell, P. H. (1969). *Scientific Basis of Drug Dependence.* (Edinburgh: Churchill) 1969
Criminal Law Review 326 (1956). *Times 8 August 1955 (J. Crim. Law*, **20**, 18)
Edwards, G. (1977). Some years on. Evolution of the 'British system'. (Cambridge: Cropwood Conference, *December*)
Fazey, C. (1979). In the heroin trap. *Guardian, 30 October*
Franks Committee (1957). *Report of the Committee on Administrative Tribunals and Enquiries*
Glancy, J. E. McA. (1972). The treatment of narcotic dependence in the United Kingdom. *Bull. Narcot.*, **24, 4**
Jeffery, C. G. (1970). *Modern Trends in Drug Dependence and Alcoholism.* (London: Butterworths)
Judson, H. F. (1974). *Heroin Addiction in Britain.* (London: Harcourt Brace Jovanovitch)
Kelly, M. G. (1972). Misuse of a morphine alternative. *J. Irish Med. Assoc.*, **65**, 482
Leech, K. (1973). *Keep the Faith Baby.* (London: SPCK)
Nyman, M. (1969). Addiction Unit – All Saints Hospital, *Br. Hosp. J. Soc. Serv. Rev., 1 August*
Phillipson, R. V. (1970) (ed.). *Modern Trends in Drug Dependence and Alcoholism.* (London: Butterworths)
Report by the Advisory Committee on Drug Dependence. (1970). *The Amphetamines and Lysergic Acid Diethylamide (LSD).* (London: HMSO)
Rolleston Committee (1926). *Departmental Committee on Morphine and Heroin Addiction.* (London: HMSO)
Spear, H. B. (1969). The growth of heroin addiction in the United Kingdom. *Br. J. Addict.*, **64**, 245
Spear, H. B. (1975). The British experience. *John Marshall J. Pract. Proc.*, **9**, 1
United Nations (1981). *Report of the International Narcotics Control Board.* (New York: United Nations)

4

The antagonist analgesic concept

J. W. Lewis

INTRODUCTION

One of the prime objectives of medical research over the past 50 years has been the discovery and development of an analgesic agent having the efficacy of morphine without the liability to abuse which characterizes the narcotics. All the opioid drugs introduced during this period have claimed superiority over morphine in terms of abuse potential. Most of them have ultimately failed to live up to the full extent of the claims made; nevertheless several widely used drugs have been less abused than morphine.

The abuse of narcotics is due to the mood-elevating effects they show in some people. These effects cause susceptible individuals to self-administer narcotics, and in so doing they become tolerant to the pleasurable effects and physically dependent on the drugs. At this point they are motivated to continue self-administration primarily to prevent the discomforting abstinence syndrome which appears only a few hours after drug administration.

Normal people when dosed with narcotics experience dysphoria, sedation and often nausea and vomiting. The addict experiences euphoria, feelings of efficiency and enhanced self-image. Sedative effects are not prominent and nausea/vomiting when experienced is described as 'pleasant sick'. In the addict the personality deficiencies giving feelings of ineptness, inefficiency, unpopularity and low personal esteem result in enhanced perception of the subjective effects of narcotics. However, these improved feelings do not apply when tolerance has been established. In the addicted state the feelings change from wellbeing and euphoria to apathy, lethargy and dysphoria (Martin, 1977).

The first morphine derivative to be introduced, in 1898, as a morphine substitute of increased effectiveness and decreased addiction liability was diacetylmorphine (heroin). It is salutary to reflect that this drug now represents by far and away the most abused opiate and is a grave sociological and public health problem. Codeine is a simple derivative of morphine (methyl ether) which has traditionally been used as an oral preparation for less severe pain and as an antidiarrhoeal and antitussive. It was shown to have morphine-like addiction liability (Himmelsbach *et al.*, 1934), but from a public health viewpoint the addiction liability of codeine was felt to be less than that of morphine. The characteristics of codeine which limited its addiction liability were its low potency and the appearance of side-effects before full morphine-like effects could be attained. The actual abuse of codeine is low, even though it is not controlled as rigorously as morphine and is more widely available as oral preparations.

In the late 1930s pethidine (meperidine in the United States) which was developed in Germany as a synthetic substitute for atropine was shown to have analgesic properties which led to its introduction as a morphine substitute lacking abuse potential. It was subsequently shown (Himmelsbach, 1942, 1943) that pethidine had addiction liability similar to morphine but nevertheless the level of actual abuse has been lower.

Methadone was introduced after the Second World War as an orally active morphine-like analgesic. It has dependence characteristics similar to those of morphine but the abstinence syndrome is less intense and slower to develop. It has found considerable use as a maintenance drug for narcotic addicts. The basis of this treatment is that subjects tolerant to the effects of one narcotic are cross-tolerant to other narcotics. Thus the methadone-maintained (tolerant) patient perceives no mood-elevation when self-administering illicit opiates. Extinguishing the effects of illicit opiates in this way enables a more stable pattern of life to be pursued with less likelihood of criminal activity and greater likelihood of useful employment.

d-Propoxyphene was introduced in 1957 as an oral analgesic for moderate pain and an alternative to codeine. Early studies (Fraser and Isbell, 1960a and b) showed that propoxyphene produced morphine-like euphoria and physical dependence but was judged to have a lower abuse potential than codeine because of its lower potency and its low toxicity threshold (nervousness, convulsions and psychoses). The actual abuse of propoxyphene is comparable to that of codeine. A particular concern about propoxyphene is that its relatively wide availability and low toxicity threshold has resulted in an increasing number of drug-related deaths.

During the study of derivatives of morphine, a group of compounds in which the *N*-methyl group of morphine was replaced by allyl or a similar group, showed the ability specifically to antagonize the effects of morphine. The most active of these compounds was nalorphine, *N*-allylnormorphine, which can bring about a dramatic recovery from the effects of narcotics overdosage. When administered to physically dependent narcotic takers it precipitates an intense withdrawal syndrome. It was shown to be an effective analgesic in man (Lasagna and Beecher, 1954) and to have an extremely low abuse potential (Wikler, Fraser and Isbell, 1953). Unfortunately, nalorphine is not clinically useful as an analgesic because of dysphoric effects including unpleasant hallucinations. Nevertheless, this discovery brought about a radical change in the direction of chemical and pharmacological thinking in the search for a safer, less abusable morphine-like agent and the search turned towards agents like nalorphine having both morphine-like (agonist) and morphine-antagonist actions. The key objective was to separate these desirable effects from the dysphoric and hallucinatory actions shown by nalorphine.

MOLECULAR PHARMACOLOGY OF MIXED AGONISTS–ANTAGONISTS

At first sight it seems to be a contradiction in terms to seek an improved morphine-like drug amongst compounds with morphine-antagonist activity. To appreciate why this is possible it is important to understand the action of such compounds at a molecular level. Theories of drug–receptor interactions, largely developed with reference to classical neurotransmitters such as acetylcholine (Ariens, Simonis and Van Rossum, 1964), can be applied to opioid drugs, particularly in the light of recent evidence supporting the existence of physiological receptors for the natural peptide opioids (Hughes *et al.*, 1975; Pert and Snyder, 1973; Simon, Hiller and Edelman, 1973; Terenius, 1973). Theoretical dose–response curves for the interaction of substances with agonist and mixed agonist–antagonist actions with a single receptor are shown in Figure 4.1. These curves demonstrate the meaning of efficacy and potency, terms which are frequently confused. A change in potency (amount of drug required to produce a particular effect), which in molecular terms is measured as receptor affinity, is reflected by a change in the positioning of the sigmoid dose–response curve with respect to the dose axis. Moving from left to right along the dose axis shows decreased affinity and hence potency. A change in drug efficacy (in molecular terms intrinsic activity), which measures the maximum response level that can be achieved by a drug (irrespective of dose), results in change of shape of the dose–response curve with the production of flatter dose–response curves by agonists having lower intrinsic activity. A number of morphine antagonists have been discovered which have high affinity for opiate receptors but zero intrinsic activity, in other words, they are 'pure' antagonists. Naloxone and naltrexone are the best known examples of this class.

The possession of both agonist and antagonist properties by low efficacy agonists (sometimes called partial agonists) can be explained by this picture. In Figure 4.2 the dose–response of a partial agonist is shown in the presence and absence of a high dose of a pure agonist. Curve *A* for the partial agonist alone becomes curve *B* in the presence of

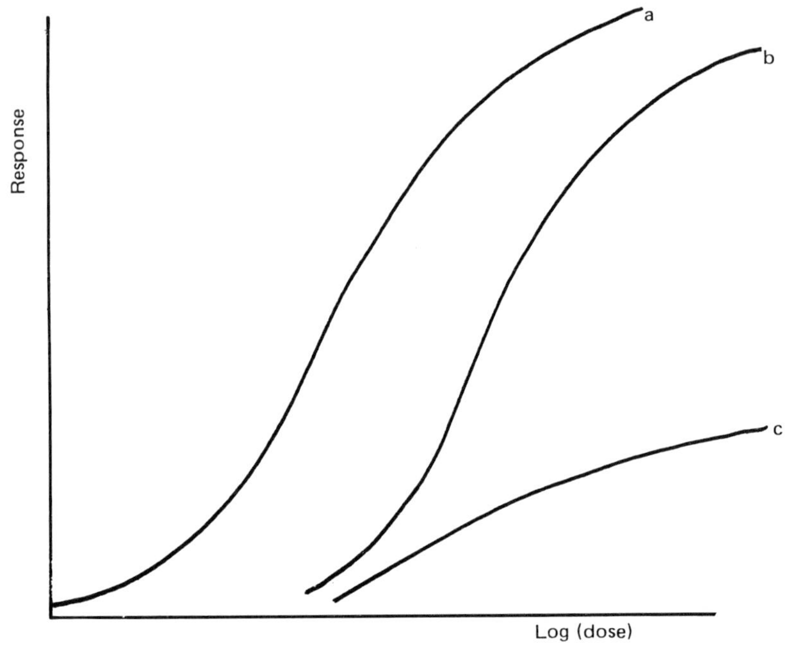

Figure 4.1 Theoretical log (dose)–response curves for the interaction of drugs with a single receptor population. Curve *a*, high-affinity pure agonist; curve *b*, low-affinity pure agonist; curve *c*, partial agonist with intrinsic activity around 0.4 (adapted from Ariens, Simonis and Van Rossum, 1964)

the agonist (morphine, for example). With increasing doses of the partial agonist, progressive displacement of the agonist occurs from the receptor with a corresponding decrease in total effect (decreased receptor output). The result is the partial reversal of the effect of the agonist by the partial agonist. The latter thus possesses the ability to antagonize the effects of a higher intrinsic activity agonist while itself possessing significant agonist activity.

The profile of nalorphine as an analgesic with morphine-antagonist properties could be explained on this single receptor model. However, some early clinical data obtained using nalorphine-morphine mixtures prompted Martin (1967) to evaluate a two-receptor model. Houde and Wallenstein (1956) had shown that low doses of nalorphine antagonized the analgesic effects of morphine while larger doses produced a lesser degree of antagonism. These data, together with information on the different abstinence syndromes associated with nalorphine and morphine in man (see below) could be better interpreted in the dual receptor model. One of these receptors (μ) is responsible for morphine's actions and the other (κ) accounts for nalorphine's agonist (analgesic) actions (Gilbert and Martin, 1976). Nalorphine was recognized as a competitive antagonist without intrinsic activity at the μ receptors; this accounts for its lack of morphine-like euphoric effects in man. These two

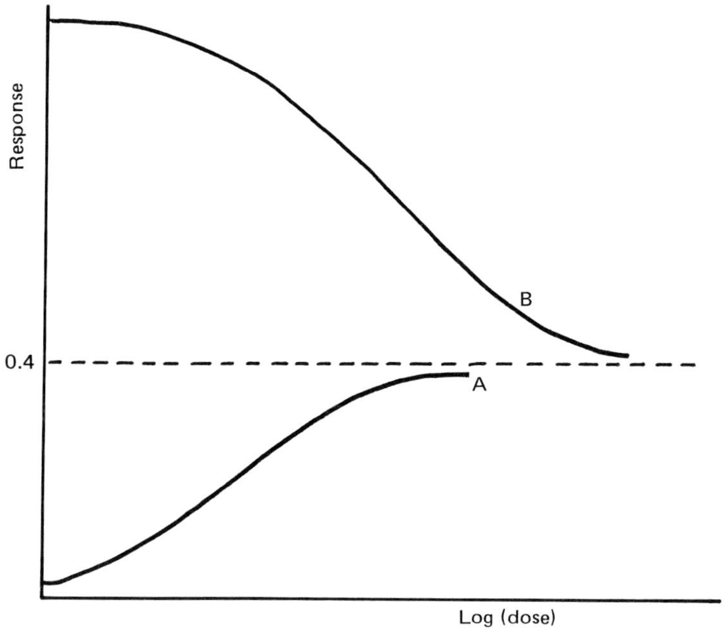

Figure 4.2 Theoretical log (dose) – response curves for the interaction of a partial agonist of intrinsic activity around 0.4 with a single receptor. Curve *A*, the partial agonist alone; curve *B*, in the presence of a saturating concentration of a second pure agonist drug. Both curves are asymptotic to the same level of response, that is, 0.4 × maximum response (adapted from Ariens, Simonis and Van Rossum, 1964)

receptors did not account for the dysphoric/hallucinogenic actions of nalorphine so Martin introduced a third receptor (σ) to account for these effects.

The many compounds that have been shown to have mixed agonist–antagonist actions can be classified in terms of Martin's three receptors. Most agents can be classified in one of two groups; the nalorphine-type possessing agonist activity at the κ and σ receptors and, predominantly, antagonism at the μ receptor, and true partial agonists of the morphine-type which possess significant but limited intrinsic activity at the μ receptor with possibly some effect at the κ but little or no action at σ receptors.

METHODS OF DETERMINING ABUSE POTENTIAL OF OPIOIDS

It was stated above that nalorphine was judged to have an extremely low abuse potential. As a result of what tests can this judgement be made and how can the results be quantitated? There are two pharmacological ways of identifying drugs with abuse potential: (1) the demonstration of reinforcing any harmful properties, and (2) demonstration of equivalence to a drug of known abuse potential. The concept of a drug having positive reinforcing characteristics is complex and related to some fundamental properties of the brain giving rise to acquisitive and avoidance behaviour and also with feeling states and associated affective behaviour. Narcotic drugs do not appear to be positively reinforcing to normal subjects (see, for example, Smith and Beecher, 1962) but are highly reinforcing to psychopaths (see Haertzen, 1966). This contrasts with the amphetamines which were shown to be universally reinforcing (Lasagna and Beecher, 1955). Reinforcing properties of narcotics are also manifest in their ability to induce tolerance and physical dependence.

From a practical standpoint the best validated method of showing abuse potential is by establishing pharmacological equivalence to a known abused narcotic. A variety of types of information serve to establish this relationship.

SELF-ADMINISTRATION TECHNIQUES

About 75% of rhesus monkeys in the drug-naive state will self-administer morphine and codeine continuously to the extent that they become physically dependent (Deneau, Yanagita and Seevers, 1969). A widely used technique which can give comparative information of the reinforcing properties of opioids is the cross self-administration procedure in which rhesus monkeys are conditioned to respond to a standard drug, usually codeine or cocaine. Access to the standard drug is limited and when a stable response rate is established, saline is substituted. The response is extinguished showing that the monkey discriminates between the reinforcing drug and saline. The monkey is then given access to the test drug and if the response rates increase *over* saline levels, the test drug is presumed to be positively reinforcing. If response rates are decreased *below* saline rates, the test drug is presumed to be aversive.

A more precise measure of reinforcing efficacy is provided by the progressive ratio test developed by Yanagita (1973). Monkeys are trained to selfadminister a standard drug, receiving one dose of drug for each 100 level presses (FR100). The standard drug is replaced by saline until the monkey reduces the number of drug injections to less than half those for the standard drug. A test drug is then substituted for saline using a FR100 schedule and self-administration is allowed. The FR ratio is doubled 24 h later, and again doubled repeatedly after a fixed number of injections. When the time intervals between injections is greater than 48 h drug seeking is said to have been extinguished, and this extinction ratio is taken as a measure of reinforcing efficacy. The extinction ratio for morphine is 12 800 (at 0.5 mg/kg i.v.) and for codeine 6400 (at 1.0 mg/kg i.v.).

SUPPRESSION OF ABSTINENCE

Studies of the ability of drugs to suppress signs of abstinence in morphine-dependent animals have been widely used as an early stage in the evaluation of abuse liability. Well-established techniques have been developed for the rat (Teiger, 1974), chronic spinalized dog (Martin *et al.*, 1974) and rhesus monkey (Deneau, 1956). The most widely used procedure for the assessment of morphine-like activity is the suppression technique in the rhesus monkey, and about 1000 drugs have been assessed at the University of Michigan using this technique.

DIRECT ADDICTION

Chronic administration of a test opioid may produce a state of physical dependence; this can be demonstrated by the abstinence syndrome which can be precipitated by a pure antagonist such as naloxone. Extensive direct addiction studies have been performed only in the rhesus monkey at the University of Michigan (Villarreal and Karbowski, 1974) and, more recently, at the Medical College of Virginia (Aceto *et al.*, 1974).

ABSTINENCE PRECIPITATION

In assessing the abuse liability of drugs with narcotic antagonist properties, additional information can be obtained by investigating the actions of a test drug in non-withdrawn, physically dependent subjects. At a particular level of physical morphine dependence a partial agonist may suppress abstinence in withdrawn subjects or precipitate abstinence in non-withdrawn subjects. By using more than one level of physical morphine dependence an estimate of the morphine-like intrinsic activity can be made.

STUDIES IN HUMAN POST-ADDICTS

Concurrently with the development of the above procedures for studying the abuse liability of opioids in animals, procedures for human experiments in prisoner ex-addicts were established at the Addiction Research Centre, Lexington, Kentucky. Substitution studies (Fraser and Isbell, 1960a and b) and direct addiction studies (Fraser *et al.*, 1961) used procedures similar to those used in the rhesus monkey. The scoring of abstinence effects was based on a scale devised by Himmelsbach (Kolb and Himmelsbach, 1938). Physical morphine dependence was established at the 240 mg/day level which was estimated to give full receptor occupation, and in direct dependence tests which lasted about 8 weeks the aim was to administer the test drug at a daily level equivalent to 240 mg morphine.

An additional set of procedures in post-addicts measured the subjective (euphoric) effects produced by test opioids and compared them with standard doses of morphine (Fraser *et al.*, 1961). Since the subjective effects of nalorphine are qualitatively different from those of morphine, when studying opioid antagonists nalorphine was often used as standard (Jasinski, Martin and Hoeldtke, 1971).

This comprehensive battery of tests has provided the information upon which the abuse liability of new agents, particularly the recently developed antagonist-analgesics, has been evaluated. The tests in human post-addicts are no longer carried out, so in future more reliance will have to be placed on the results of animal tests.

PROFILES OF ANTAGONIST-ANALGESICS

NALORPHINE

The human pharmacology of nalorphine was studied by Isbell and his collaborators at the Addiction Research Centre. Single doses as well as chronic administration of nalorphine produced dysphoric effects (Isbell, 1956; Wikler, Fraser and Isbell, 1953). In a later study (Haertzen, 1970) using a 40-item questionnaire designed to distinguish opiates from other psychotropic agents, nalorphine produced no significant changes in euphoria-related items, but significant effects in measures of psychotomimetic effects and those associated with sedation, drunkenness and disorientation. Nalorphine precipitated abstinence in morphine-dependent subjects (Wikler, Fraser and Isbell, 1953).

The direct addiction study of nalorphine was undertaken by Martin and Gorodetsky (1965) at a dose of 240 mg/day for 32 days. Withdrawal of nalorphine produced many signs similar to those observed in morphine abstinence such as rhinorrhoea, yawning, lacrimation, chills, diarrhoea, loss of appetite and body weight, but there were also significant differences in that blood pressure and respiratory rate were only slightly increased, and at early times following withdrawal a sensation in the head was experienced which was described as electric shocks or lightheadedness. Itching was also a feature of nalorphine abstinence. A most important difference between the nalorphine and morphine abstinence syndromes was that nalorphine subjects were not concerned about their symptoms and did not seek drugs (narcotics) to relieve them. The conclusion from these studies was that nalorphine was lacking in abuse potential and this has been borne out in practice.

BENZOMORPHANS

Following the discovery of the narcotic antagonist properties of nalorphine, other *N*-substituents related to the allyl group where shown also to produce antagonists. One of the most important of these groups is the cyclopropylmethyl group which was first incorporated into codeine by von Braun, Kuhn and Siffiqui (1926). Subsequently, synthetic structures simpler than morphine were recognized as having useful analgesic potential. Notable among these were the benzomorphans and this chemical group was widely explored by Archer *et al.* (1964) as a source of antagonist-analgesics. Two of these compounds became of clinical importance: pentazocine and cyclazocine.

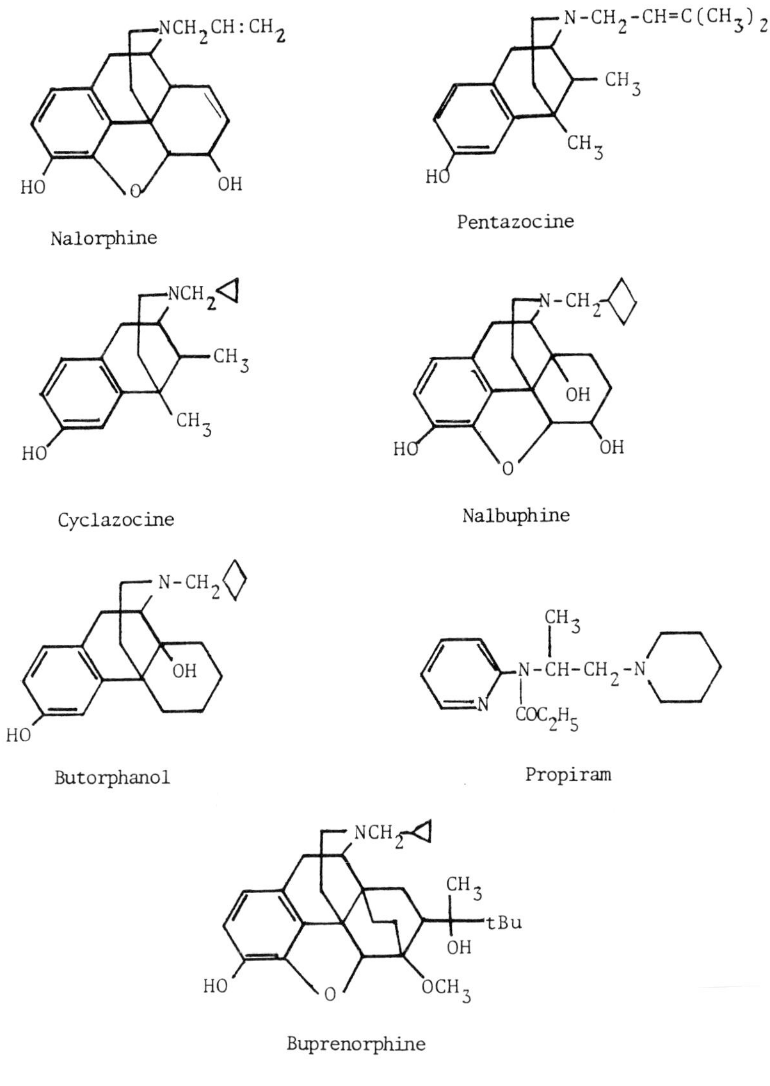

Chemical structure of antagonist-analgesics

Cyclazocine

Of the two benzomorphans selected for clinical study cyclazocine was by far the more potent both as an analgesic (approximately 40 times more than morphine) and as a morphine-antagonist (five times more than nalorphine) in man. As its profile is quite similar to that of nalorphine it too has not been introduced as an analgesic. Martin *et al.* (1965) studied the human pharmacology of cyclazocine in post-addicts. The subjective effects of single doses of cyclazocine at lower doses bore resemblance to those of morphine but larger doses produced psychotomimetic effects and sedation. The abstinence syndrome following chronic administration was nalorphine-like with no drug-seeking behaviour.

In self-administration studies in non-dependent monkeys, cyclazocine was shown to be aversive (Hoffmeister and Wuttke, 1973). Following the observation that nalorphine and cyclazocine produced a non-morphine-like abstinence syndrome in man, it was shown that different abstinence syndromes were produced in rhesus monkeys by morphine and cyclazocine (Villarreal, 1972). The cyclazocine abstinence syndrome was characterized by yawning and scratching which are among the mild characteristics of morphine abstinence in monkeys.

Pentazocine

Pentazocine was the first antagonist-analgesic to be introduced into clinical practice for the relief of moderate to severe pain. It is a less potent analgesic than morphine (approximately 0.25 times) (Houde, 1979), and also only a weak antagonist (approximately 0.02 times nalorphine) (Jasinski, Martin and Hoeldtke, 1970). Pentazocine produces subjective effects in man which resemble both morphine and nalorphine. In single-dose studies, subcutaneous doses of 40 mg or less produced signs and symptoms that were indistinguishable from those of modest doses (10 mg) of morphine, whereas at higher doses ($\geqslant$ 60 mg) the effects of pentazocine were predominantly nalorphine-like (Jasinski, Martin and Hoeldtke, 1970). Pentazocine precipitated abstinence in morphine-dependent subjects stabilized at a high morphine dose (240 mg/day). It did not suppress abstinence in lower-dose, withdrawn, morphine-dependent subjects (60 mg/day). However, in 30 mg/day dependent subjects pentazocine does suppress abstinence (Jasinski, 1977). In direct addiction studies in subjects stabilized on doses of pentazocine greater than 500 mg/day, abrupt withdrawal produced a mild abstinence syndrome with both morphine-like and nalorphine-like features. Of significance was the request for drugs to relieve the pentazocine abstinence syndrome. Naloxone but not nalorphine precipitated a moderately severe abstinence syndrome in these subjects (Jasinski, Martin and Hoeldtke, 1970).

Pentazocine is self-administered by drug-naive monkeys (Yanagita, 1973) whereas it is aversive (negative reinforcing) in morphine-dependent monkeys (Schlicting and Hoffmeister, 1971). The aversive behaviour is presumably an antecedent of precipitated withdrawal. In the progressive ratio test Yanagita (1975) reported extinction ratios for pentazocine (0.25 mg/kg i.v.) of 6400 in saline pretreated monkeys and 3200 in pentazocine-dependent animals. The corresponding figures for morphine (0.5 mg/kg i.v.) were 6400 and 12 800. Thus in non-dependent monkeys pentazocine is as reinforcing as morphine but in the dependent state pentazocine is less reinforcing.

Pentazocine precipitated abstinence in withdrawn monkeys dependent on 12 mg/kg per day of morphine. However, in monkeys at a lower level (1.2 mg/kg per day) pentazocine suppressed abstinence (Yanagita, 1975). In direct addiction studies in monkeys pentazocine produced only a mild abstinence syndrome on abrupt withdrawal (Yanagita, 1975).

The overall profile of pentazocine as both like morphine and nalorphine emerges from these studies. In receptor terms it would appear that pentazocine has low affinity and intrinsic activity at the morphine (μ) receptor, and rather higher intrinsic activity at the $\varkappa$ and σ receptors.

As an alternative to the Addiction Research Centre procedures for evaluating abuse potential in prisoners, Schuster, Smith and Jaffe (1971) investigated the reinforcing efficacy of codeine, methadone and pentazocine as oral preparations in narcotic addicts. In the first experiment codeine and pentazocine over a 4-day trial were made available to heroin abusers at the end of a detoxification period. Subjects were maintained in hospital and placebo control was used. Both pentazocine and codeine groups took about 85% of the available administrations compared with 50% for placebo. In a second experiment, in outpatient addicts who were awaiting enrolment in a state rehabilitation programme, methadone (40 mg/day), codeine (400 mg/day) and pentazocine (400 mg/day) were compared with placebo. For 5 days treatments were available on a daily basis and a modest attendance fee ($2) was given to volunteers as expenses. At the end of 5 days subjects were told that the experiment would last another 5 days but the $2 expenses would not be available. In the first 5 days the frequency of clinic attendance of subjects receiving methadone (68%) and codeine (57%) was higher than those receiving pentazocine (39%) and placebo (49%). In the second 5-day period the difference was even more marked. The finishing to starting percentages were methadone 32, codeine 35, placebo 18 and pentazocine 13%.

There are thus significant differences in the results of the two experiments. In the hospital, when only a short walk is necessary to obtain drugs, and when there were no other sources of drugs, pentazocine and codeine were equally attractive to the addict. In the second study they were required to travel to the hospital and spend about an hour there on various tests. In this situation the relatively weak reinforcing effects of pentazocine were well demonstrated. Another factor was that the hospitalized subjects had been detoxified whereas a significant proportion of the outpatients were physically dependent as judged by urine morphine levels. In these subjects pentazocine was likely to be aversive as it was in physically dependent monkeys.

Pentazocine was introduced into clinical practice in 1967 as an analgesic not subject to narcotic controls. Reports of its abuse appeared a few years later (Inciardi and Chambers, 1971). Abuse was limited to the medical community and patients (Swanson, Weddige and Morse, 1973), and street abuse was unpopular until recently. Chronic parenteral abuse of pentazocine injections may result in severe skin ulceration, muscle fibrosis, and vasculitis (Podilla *et al.*, 1979). During the past 5 years pentazocine has been found as a drug on the streets where it is combined with tripelennamine. Tablets of the two drugs are dissolved and injected intravenously. This combination, known as 'T's and Blues', was first used on the streets of Chicago but has since been reported in other US cities (Showalter, 1980). Tripelennamine has for many years been abused in combination with heroin or morphine. The reason for its attraction to street addicts is uncertain though it had been tried as a treatment for morphine withdrawal in the 1940s. The combination of the two drugs appears to eliminate the undesirable effects of the drugs alone.

In order to estimate the relative level of abuse of pentazocine when compared with other opioids, the hardest available data is provided in the information collected in the United States through the Drug Abuse Warning Network (DAWN). These data refer to non-medical uses and drug-related deaths collected from emergency rooms, inpatient units in non-federal short-term general hospitals, county medical examiners or county coroners and crisis intervention centres. The results for 1973–75 are shown in Table 4.1 and the continued trend has been shown up to 1976–77 (Jasinski, 1977, 1979).

Table 4.1 *Relative levels of abuse of opioid drugs in the United States*

Drug	*DAWN mentions 1973–75* (A)	*Estimated relative availability*			*Relative abuse* (A/B)
		Aggregated US 1973 production (kg)	*Potency (parenteral)*	*Morphine equivalence* (kg) (B)	
Morphine	3760	535	1	535	7.0
Codeine	4343	32 564	0.1	3256	1.3
Meperidine	1689	16 292	0.1	1629	1.0
Methadone	9864	3339	1	3339	3.0
d-Propoxyphene	9692	88 120	0.07	6168	1.6
Pentazocine	1832	10 087	0.3	3026	0.6

Propoxyphene and codeine, which are less abused than morphine despite being less strictly controlled, are available only in oral forms and toxic symptoms limit dosage levels. These factors play a part in limiting their abuse but, especially in the case of propoxyphene, lethal overdosage is a major problem (Wetli and Bednorczyk, 1980). Pentazocine which is available in intravenous as well as oral form is less abused than any of the other drugs. The comparison between pentazocine and propoxyphene is significant since they are subject to the same relatively low level of control in the United States (Schedule 4).

As a clinical analgesic pentazocine at its usable limit of 60 mg seems to be as effective as 15 mg morphine (Houde, 1974) though the adequacy of analgesia and the occurrence of unwanted effects seems to be less predictable than with morphine (Brogden, Speight and Avery, 1973). Pentazocine is generally felt to be contraindicated in angina and myocardial infarction in that it may aggravate myocardial ischaemia by increasing myocardial oxygen consumption. Psychotomimetic effects are a problem with pentazocine more especially in patients with severe chronic pain and in those who have previously received significant quantities of narcotics (Houde, 1974).

In summary, to a reasonable extent pentazocine lived up to the hopes of lower abuse than morphine with good analgesia. However, its shortcomings were clear so that the search for other antagonist analgesics continued in the benzomorphan and other areas of opioid chemistry. From the 14-hydroxymorphine series nalbuphine was developed and from the 14-hydroxymorphinan series, butorphanol.

Nalbuphine

The pharmacological profile of nalbuphine like that of pentazocine shows elements of both morphine-like and nalorphine-like activity. An important quantitative difference is that it is less psychotomimetic than pentazocine in man. In single doses in post-addicts nalbuphine (8 mg) produced subjective effects and miosis equivalent to morphine (10 mg). Increasing the dose of nalbuphine to 72 mg produced little increase in the level of morphine-like effects and only minimal psychotomimetic effects (Jasinski and Mansky, 1972). Nalbuphine precipitated abstinence in subjects dependent on morphine 60 mg/day, whereas at the 30 mg/day level nalbuphine suppressed abstinence in withdrawn subjects. Chronic administration of nalbuphine (203 mg/day) produced physical dependence similar to that of pentazocine with a mild to moderate abstinence syndrome being produced which resulted in requests for drug to assuage it (Jasinski and Mansky, 1972). During this direct addiction study nalbuphine did not produce any mood elevation, which was in sharp contrast to the earlier study of Elliott, Navarro and Nomoff (1970) who found that addicts consistently identified nalbuphine as 'dope' over a 7-day trial during which a low level of physical dependence was established. The difference between the two results almost certainly arises from the different dose levels employed. In Jasinski's study at over 200 mg/day the incursion of nalorphine-like effects will have negated morphine-like euphoria, whereas Elliott's study was conducted at 40 mg/day (4 × 10 mg). In single doses 10 mg nalbuphine was more reliably identified as 'dope' than was morphine by Elliott's subjects.

In rhesus monkeys trained to self-administer codeine, nalbuphine maintained response rates above saline levels but below those for codeine and propoxyphene (Woods, 1978). In a direct addiction study in monkeys naloxone precipitated a morphine-like abstinence syndrome of high intensity.

From these human and animal studies it emerges that nalbuphine is pentazocine-like but the balance of morphine-like to nalbuphine-like effects is different. In receptor terms, at the μ and κ receptors the intrinsic activity of nalbuphine and pentazocine appear similar but with nalbuphine having higher affinity. The lower affinity of nalbuphine at the σ receptor accounts for the greater separation of morphine-like and dysphoric effects.

Nalbuphine was introduced as an analgesic in the United States in 1979. In clinical trials it was shown to be about equipotent with morphine, and five times more potent and with a somewhat longer duration of action than pentazocine. In a comparative trial against pentazocine in cancer patients who had undergone surgery seven of the 27 patients who received 60 mg pentazocine experienced psychotomimetic effects whereas only three of 58 patients who received 10 or 20 mg nalbuphine had similar experiences (Houde *et al.*, 1976).

Butorphanol

Butorphanol is another drug with essentially pentazocine-like profile which was introduced in 1978 in the United States. In studies at the Addiction Research Centre, butorphanol produced morphine-like responses in modest doses but nalorphine-like effects at higher doses. The separation of these effects was greater than with pentazocine but less than with nalbuphine. In subjects dependent upon 60 mg/day morphine, butorphanol neither precipitated nor suppressed abstinence when subjects were made abstinent. In the direct addiction study naloxone precipitated a moderately severe abstinence syndrome, and on abrupt withdrawal a somewhat milder syndrome developed which had some nalorphine-like features, but with a limited level of drug-seeking behaviour (Jasinski, 1977).

In self-administration studies in codeine-trained rhesus monkeys, butorphanol maintained injection rates above saline but below codeine (Woods, 1977). As in man, butorphanol did not precipitate abstinence in morphine-dependent rhesus monkeys and in a direct dependence study in monkeys naloxone precipitated a moderately severe abstinence syndrome; the syndrome following abrupt withdrawal was graded as moderate (Woods *et al.*, 1980).

Thus butorphanol demonstrates a pentazocine-like profile with higher receptor affinity than pentazocine. In clinical trials this profile has been confirmed (Houde, 1979).

PARTIAL AGONISTS OF THE MORPHINE-TYPE

The actions of the drugs so far described cannot be explained using a one-receptor model – they all appear to have some affinity for all three of Martin's receptors, μ, κ and σ. There is a group of drugs whose actions can be accounted for by their action at the μ receptor where they are partial agonists. The main difference between the clinical pharmacological profiles of the two types of analgesics is the lack of dysphoria and psychotomimetic effects shown by the partial agonists. The two morphine-like partial agonists which have been most investigated are propiram and buprenorphine.

PROPIRAM

In single-dose studies in post-addicts propiram was shown to have a morphine-like profile though at high doses some dysphoric effects were noted. These were not identified as nalorphine-like. In subjects dependent upon 240 mg/day of morphine, propiram precipitated abstinence but only at high dose (potency 0.005 × nalorphine) whereas at the 60 mg morphine/day in withdrawn subjects propiram suppressed abstinence. Thus the intrinsic activity at the μ receptor was greater than that of pentazocine, nalbuphine and butorphanol, all of which failed to suppress abstinence in 60 mg/day morphine-dependent subjects. In the direct addiction study nalorphine precipitated an opiate-like withdrawal syndrome and in this respect the higher intrinsic activity of propiram was again demonstrated since the pentazocine-like agents in direct addiction studies showed no response to nalorphine, requiring the pure antagonist naloxone to precipitate abstinence. From these studies it was concluded that propiram may have a lower abuse potential than propoxyphene and codeine but greater than that of pentazocine (Jasinski, Martin and Hoedtke, 1971).

Propiram appears to have a similar profile to pentazocine in self-administration studies in monkeys. In naive or codeine-trained monkeys it is positively reinforcing with an extinction ratio of 3200 in Yanagita's tests (Jasinski, 1977). It is negatively reinforcing in morphine-dependent monkeys (Schlicting and Hoffmeister, 1971) and precipitates abstinence in highly dependent monkeys. Like pentazocine it suppresses abstinence in monkeys withdrawn from low-level dependence (Yanagita, 1975).

In clinical trials propiram was shown to be an effective analgesic with about one-tenth of morphine's potency by the intramuscular route (Forrest *et al.*, 1972). It is particularly effective as an oral product with an onset of action comparable with that of intramuscular morphine (Houde *et al.*, 1977). In all these studies side-effects were morphine-like with no evidence of dysphoria or psychotomimetic reactions. Despite this attractive clinical analgesic profile propiram has not yet been introduced into clinical practice. No doubt one of the major reasons for this is that the WHO has classified propiram as a narcotic and placed it under strict legal control.

BUPRENORPHINE

Unlike all the agents so far considered buprenorphine possesses a chemical structure significantly more complex than that of morphine. It was first identified as a partial morphine-like agonist from elegant studies in the chronic spinal dog by Martin *et al.* (1976) who showed that buprenorphine partially suppressed abstinence in withdrawn morphine-dependent dogs as well as precipitating abstinence in non-withdrawn animals. The slopes of the dose–response curves for both of these actions were shallower than for the standard agonist propoxyphene and antagonist naloxone respectively. Buprenorphine precipitated abstinence in morphine-dependent rhesus monkeys (Swain and Seevers, 1975) and failed to suppress abstinence in withdrawn, morphine-dependent monkeys (Yanagita, private communication). In direct addiction studies in rhesus monkeys (Swain and Seevers, 1975) and patas monkeys (Cowan, 1974) naloxone failed to precipitate abstinence and no abstinence signs were observed following abrupt withdrawal.

In rhesus monkeys trained to self-administer codeine, buprenorphine maintained response levels well above saline but less than codeine (Woods, 1977). Buprenorphine was self-administered by a drug-naive monkey (Mello, Bree and Mendelson, 1981). In a continuous self-administration study four monkeys self-administered between 1.07 and 3.3 mg/kg per day without showing marked depression or stimulation; when saline was substituted for the drug, behaviour remained normal and no withdrawal signs were observed (Yanagita, private communication). In the progressive ratio test buprenorphine was compared with pentazocine in a crossover experiment in four monkeys, using two doses of each drug. With pentazocine all monkeys recorded higher ratios for the larger dose (0.25 mg/kg by injection), whereas for buprenorphine three animals showed higher scores at 15 μg/kg by injection and only one at 60 μg/kg by injection. It was concluded that buprenorphine may have lower psychological dependence potential than pentazocine (Yanagita, private communication).

The clinical pharmacological studies undertaken by Jasinski, Pevnick and Griffith (1978) in post-addicts confirmed the profile which had been established in animal studies. In single-dose studies it produced morphine-like subjective effects and was estimated to be 25 to 50 times more potent than morphine. In two out of three studies there was a negative dose–response but the impression was that the ceiling to the morphine-like effects was at a dose level corresponding to 20–30 mg of morphine; no nalorphine-like dysphoric effects were detected. In the direct addiction study naloxone failed to precipitate any abstinence syndrome and on abrupt withdrawal, only 14 days later were any clinically significant effects seen. Buprenorphine's profile in direct addiction studies is therefore different from the other agents in that the abstinence syndrome in the 2 or 3 days following abrupt withdrawal, which is the reinforcing aspect of physical dependence, is missing following chronic administration of buprenorphine.

It is surprising that a drug with such a strong morphinomimetic profile should appear not to produce physical dependence. The reason for this apparent anomaly probably lies in the unusual receptor kinetics of buprenorphine. The rate at which a drug leaves its receptor site when challenged with an antagonist or on abrupt withdrawal is important in determining the severity of the abstinence syndrome produced. In studies both *in vivo* and *in vitro* (Rance and Dickens, 1978) it has been shown that buprenorphine dissociates extremely slowly from opiate receptors in the rat brain. This phenomenon results in homeostatic control of the biochemical imbalances which occur on withdrawal of opioid from the receptor and which are responsible for the excitatory withdrawal syndrome (Lewis and Rance, 1979).

Confirmation that buprenorphine, in common with other opioids, does indeed produce physical dependence was sought by Dum, Bläsig and Herz (1981). Recognizing that the manifestation of physical dependence – the abstinence syndrome – is inhibited by the unusual receptor kinetics of buprenorphine, they replaced buprenorphine with morphine at the end of multidose buprenorphine treatment in rats. In this way the effects of the buprenorphine treatment would be demonstrated by the removal from the receptor of a drug with normal kinetics. Using a single morphine injection and high-dose naloxone challenge 1 hour later, moderate abstinence was precipitated. It is, however, doubtful whether the morphine had a significant effect in this experiment since it was administered 12 hours after the last dose of buprenorphine, so that naloxone challenge occurred 13 hours after buprenorphine; challenge with naloxone 12 hours after the last buprenorphine administration without morphine intervention produced abstinence of similar intensity. Nevertheless, evidence was obtained that the organic and biochemical changes which occur in the establishment of physical dependence do indeed occur with buprenorphine.

Reference was made above (p. 82) to the use of methadone as a maintenance drug for opiate addicts. An alternative treatment procedure involves blockade of the effects of opiates by chronic treatment with narcotic antagonists. Cyclazocine and the 'pure' antagonists naloxone and, especially, naltrexone, have been used in this paradigm. Behind it lies the theory that by blocking the effects of opiates the reinforcing properties of opiates to the addict would be extinguished. Buprenorphine has the characteristics of both methadone and naltrexone which suggested that it might be a useful treatment for addicts. Accordingly in the primary addiction study of buprenorphine at the Addiction Research Centre, Jasinski, Pevnick and Griffith (1978) challenged their subjects with large single doses of morphine and showed that the euphoric effects were blocked. In a similar experiment Mello and Mendelson (1980) showed that chronically dosed buprenorphine blocked the effects of heroin in addicts.

In both these studies, subjects stabilized on high doses of buprenorphine received morphine or heroin. There was no evidence of any abstinence brought about by the challenges so that there appear to be few practical consequences of the effects reported in rats by Dum, Bläsig and Herz (1981), and described above.

Buprenorphine has undergone extensive clinical evaluation, mostly in the treatment of post-operative and intractable (primarily cancer) pain, and was introduced in injection form in the United Kingdom in 1978. By injection it is about 30 times more potent than morphine (Houde *et al.*, 1977) and many studies have shown that it has a longer duration of action than morphine. However, this characteristic is more demonstrable when buprenorphine is used to prevent pain following surgery (Kay, 1978) than when it is used to counteract established pain (Houde *et al.*, 1977).

In analgesic anaesthesia, De Castro and Parmentier (1976) found that doses of 0.4–1.8 mg buprenorphine produced analgesia adequate for minor surgical procedures when reinforced with nitrous oxide or flunitrazepam but it was generally unsatisfactory as the sole agent. They also showed that buprenorphine could act as an antagonist of fentanyl used in the same procedure, giving good analgesia in the post-operative period.

Buprenorphine is up to 20 times less potent by the oral route than by injection but it is well absorbed sublingually and by this route 0.4 mg has been estimated to give analgesia equivalent to 0.3 mg intramuscularly (Edge, Cooper and Morgan, 1979). In the treatment of chronic cancer pain sublingual buprenorphine in doses up to 4.8 mg/day has been shown to provide good pain relief, and where necessary withdrawal of drug has been achieved without the appearance of abstinence effects (Adriaensen and Van de Walle, 1976).

One of the potential advantages of partial agonists (and nalorphine-like agents) is that, having a ceiling to their agonist effects, they should be safer in terms of respiratory depression. In the case of buprenorphine it has been demonstrated in animal studies that for both antinociceptive and respiratory depressant effects the dose–response curve is bell-shaped with high doses producing less effect than the intermediate doses that produce maximum effect (Rance, 1979). The position of the ceiling effect in man has not been demonstrated unequivocally but extremely high doses (7 mg i.v.) have been administered to some post-operative patients with no sign of respiratory depression (Budd, private communication).

SUMMARY AND CONCLUSIONS

Following the demonstration that nalorphine was a clinically effective analgesic with negligible abuse liability, the mixed agonist-antagonists have been of prime interest as potential substitutes for morphine. Two subclasses of these agents have been investigated. Each has morphine-like actions at low doses; they differ in whether or not nalorphine-like effects are shown at higher doses. The possession of some nalorphinic character by pentazocine, nalbuphine and butorphanol limits their euphorigenic actions in single doses and gives a character to the physical dependence produced on chronic dosing in which less drug-seeking behaviour is shown in the abstinence syndrome. The true morphine-like partial agonists, of which buprenorphine is the only example available in medical practice, are free from nalorphine-like psychotomimetic effects which makes them more acceptable as analgesics but clearly establishes their direct pharmacological relationship to morphine. However, buprenorphine is a unique agent in that it does not produce the manifestations of physical dependence – the abstinence syndrome – so that this aspect of opiate reinforcement is extremely weak.

These characteristics of the antagonist-analgesics have emerged from a thorough study of their abuse liability in animal and human models, from which it has been concluded that all four agents are less likely to be abused than any opiate agonist including codeine and propoxyphene. Only pentazocine has been available long enough for meaningful statistics to be available, but in its case it would appear to be true that it is less abused than codeine and propoxyphene. It has to be recognized that the actual frequency of abuse of any drug depends on legal controls, the overall availability of the drug and the preparations in which it is marketed, knowledge of its actions, and customs and fads among the drug-abusing population, as well as its pharmacological profile which is the only subject for abuse liability evaluation.

From the viewpoint of their clinical efficacy as analgesics the antagonist-analgesics should theoretically have ceilings to their agonist actions, which in certain circumstances should make them less effective than agonists such as morphine. However, in most clinical studies of analgesics the effect level at which drugs are being compared is only defined by the doses of a standard drug. Thus most studies have lacked the sensitivity to show differences in slope of dose–response curves and ceiling effects, and limitations of analgesic efficacy for the antagonist-analgesics have not been clearly demonstrated. They are for most practical purposes able to substitute for morphine in the treatment of moderate to severe pain.

The search for a morphine substitute of negligible abuse liability which has commanded so much scientific commitment over the past 50 years has been a commendable therapeutic objective but in view of the overwhelming abuse of heroin it seems unlikely ever to solve the major sociological problem. Nevertheless from within the class of antagonist-analgesics, several agents have been developed with significant advantages over morphine and one of them, buprenorphine, may also become an important agent in the treatment of opiate dependence.

REFERENCES

Aceto, M. D., Harris, L. S., Balster, R. L. and Dewey, W. L. In: *Minutes of Thirty-Sixth Annual Scientific Meeting, Committee on Problems of Drug Dependence*, Mexico City, pp. 77–87

Adriaensen, H. and Van de Walle, J. (1976). *Acta Anaesth. Belg.*, **27**, 183

Archer, S., Albertson, N. F., Harris, L. S., Pierson, A. K. and Bird, J. G. (1964). *J. Med. Chem.*, **7**, 123–127

Ariens, E. J., Simonis, A. M. and Van Rossum, J. M. (1964). *Molecular Pharmacology: The Mode of Action of Biologically Active Compounds*. (New York: Academic Press)

Brogden, R. N., Speight, T. M. and Avery, G. S. (1973). *Drugs*, **5**, 6–91
De Castro, J. and Parmentier, P. (1976). In Huzler, E. (ed.) *Anaesthesiology, Proceedings of the Sixth World Congress of Anaesthesiology*, Mexico City, pp. 103–105. (Amersterdam: Excerpta Medica International Series No. 399)
Cowan, A. (1974). In: *Narcotic Antagonists. Advances in Biochemical Psychopharmacology. Vol. 8*. Braude, M. C., Harris, L. S., May, E. L., Smith, J. P. and Villarreal, J. E. (eds.) (New York: Raven Press)
Deneau, G. A. (1956). Dessertation for PhD degree, University of Michigan
Deneau, G., Yanagita, T. and Seevers, M. H. (1969). *Psychopharmacologia (Berl.)*, **16**, 30
Dum, J., Bläsig, J. and Herz, A. (1981). *Eur. J. Pharmacol.*, **70**, 293
Edge, W. G., Cooper, G. M. and Morgan, M. (1979). *Anaesthesia*, **34**, 463
Elliott, H. W., Navarro, G. and Nomoff, N. (1970). *J. Med.*, **1**, 74
Forrest, W. H., Brown, C. R., Schrott, P. and Teutsch, G. (1972). *J. Clin. Pharmacol.*, **12**, 440
Fraser, H. F. and Isbell, H. (1960a), *Bull. Narcot.*, **12**, 9
Fraser, H. F. and Isbell, H. (1960b). *Bull. Narcot.*, **12**, 15
Fraser, H. F., Van Horn, G. D., Martin, W. R., Wolbach, A. B. and Isbell, H. (1961). *J. Pharmacol. Exp. Ther.*, **133**, 371
Gilbert, P. E. and Martin, W. R. (1976). *J. Pharmacol. Exp. Ther.*, **198**, 66
Haertzen, C. A. (1966). *Psychol. Rep.*, **18**, 163
Haertzen, C. A. (1970). *Psychopharmacologia (Berl.)*, **18**, 366
Himmelsbach, C. K. (1934). *J. Am. Med. Assoc.*, **103**, 1420
Himmelsbach, C. K. (1942). *J. Pharmacol. Exp. Ther.*, **75**, 64
Himmelsbach, C. K. (1943). *J. Pharmacol. Exp. Ther.*, **79**, 5
Hoffmeister, F. and Wuttke, W. (1973). *Psychopharmacologia (Berl.)*, **33**, 247
Houde, R. W. and Wallenstein, S. L. (1956). *Fed. Proc.*, **15**, 440
Houde, R. W. (1974). In Bonica, J. J. (ed.) *Advances in Neurology. Vol. 4*, pp. 527–536. (New York: Raven Press)
Houde, R. W., Wallenstein, S. L., Rogers, A. and Kaiko, R. F. In Bonica, J. J. and Albe-Fessard, D. (eds.), *Advances in Pain Research and Therapy, Vol. 1*, pp. 647–751 (New York: Raven Press)
Houde, R. W., Wallenstein, S. L., Rogers, A. and Kaiko, R. F. (1977). In: *Minutes of Thirty-Ninth Scientific Meeting, Committee on Problems of Drug Dependence, Inc.*, pp. 183–216
Houde, R. W. (1979). *Br. J. Clin. Pharmacol.*, **7**, 297S
Hughes, J., Smith, T. W., Kosterlitz, H. W., Fothergill, L. A., Morgan, B. A. and Morris, H. R. (1975). *Nature (London)*, **258**, 577
Isbell, H. (1956). *Fed. Proc.*, **15**, 442
Inciardi, J. A. and Chambers, C. D. (1971). *N.Y. State J. Med.*, **71**, 1727
Jasinski, D. R., Martin, W. R. and Hoeldtke, R. D. (1970). *Clin. Pharmacol. Ther.*, **11**, 385
Jasinski, D. R., Martin, W. R. and Hoeldtke, R. D. (1971). *Clin. Pharmacol. Ther.*, **12**, 613
Jasinski, D. R. and Mansky, P. (1972). *Clin. Pharmacol. Ther.*, **13**, 78
Jasinski, D. R., Pevnick, J. S. and Griffith, J. D. (1978). *Arch. Gen. Psychiatry*, **35**, 501
Jasinski, D. R. (1977). In Martin, W. R. (ed.) *Drug Addiction I*. pp. 197–258 (Berlin, Heidelberg and New York: Springer-Verlag)
Jasinski, D. R. (1979). *Br. J. Clin. Pharmacol.*, **7**, 287S
Kay, B. (1978). *Br. J. Anaesth.*, **50 (6)**, 605
Kolb, L. and Himmelsbach, C. K. (1938). *Am. J. Psychiatry*, **94**, 759
Lasagna, L. and Beecher, H. K. (1954). *J. Pharmacol. Exp. Ther.*, **112**, 356

Lewis, J. W. and Rance, M. J. (1979). *Pharmaceut. J.*, **222**, 61
Martin, W. R. and Gorodetsky, C. W. (1965). *J. Pharmacol. Exp. Ther.*, **150**, 437
Martin, W. R., Fraser, H. F., Gorodetsky, C. W. and Rosenberg, D. E. (1965). *J. Pharmacol. Exp. Ther.*, **150**, 426
Martin, W. R. (1967). *Pharmacol. Rev.*, **19**, 463
Martin, W. R. (1977). In Martin, W. R. (ed.) *Drug Addiction I.* pp. 3–40 (Berlin, Heidelberg and New York: Springer-Verlag)
Martin, W. R., Eades, C. G., Thompson, W. O., Thompson, J. A. and Flanary, H. G. (1974). *J. Pharmacol. Exp. Ther.*, **189**, 759
Martin, W. R., Eades, C. G. Thompson, J. A., Huppler, R. E. and Gilbert, P. E. (1976). *J. Pharmacol. Exp. Ther.*, **197**, 517
Mello, N. K. and Mendelson, J. H. (1980). *Science*, **207**, 657
Mello, N. K., Bree, M. P. and Mendelson, J. H. (1981). *Pharmacol. Biochem. Behav.* (In Press)
Pert, C. B. and Snyder, S. (1973). *Science*, **179**, 1011
Podilla, R. S., Becker, L. F., Hoffman, H. *et al.* (1978). *Arch. Dermatol.*, **115**, 975
Rance, M. J. and Dickens, J. M. (1978). In Van Ree, J. M. and Terenius, L. (ed.) *Characteristics and Function of Opioids.* pp. 65–66. (Amsterdam: North Holland)
Rance, M. J. (1979). *Br. J. Clin. Pharmacol.*, *7*, 281S
Schuster, C. R., Smith, B. B. and Jaffe, J. H. (1971). *Arch. Gen. Psychiatry*, **24**, 359
Schlicting, U. U. and Hoffmeister, F. (1971). *Naunyn-Schmiedebergs Arch. Exp. Pathol. Pharmacol.*, **Suppl. to Vol. 270**, R123
Showalter, C. V. (1980). *J. Am. Med. Assoc.*, **244**, 1224
Simon, E. J., Hiller, J. M. and Edelman, I. (1973). *Proc. Natl. Acad. Sci., USA*, **70**, 1947
Smith, G. M. and Beecher, H. K. (1962). *J. Pharmacol. Exp. Ther.*, **136**, 47
Swain, H. H. and Seevers, M. H. (1975). In *Minutes of Thirty-Seventh Scientific Meeting. Committee on Problems of Drug Dependence*, pp. 773–795
Swanson, D. W., Weddige, R. L. and Morse, R. M. (1973). *Mayo Clin. Proc.*, **48**, 85–93
Teiger, D. G. (1974). *J. Pharmacol. Exp. Ther.*, **190**, 408
Terenius, L. (1973). *Acta Pharmacol. Toxicol.*, **32**, 317
Von Braun, J., Kuhn, M. and Siffiqui, S. (1926). *Ber. Dtsch. Chem. Ges.*, **59**, 1081
Van Felsinger, J. M., Lasagna, L. and Beecher, H. K. (1955). *J. Am. Med. Assoc.*, **157**, 1113
Villarreal, J. E. (1972). In Kosterlitz, H. W., Collier, H. O. J. and Villarreal, J. E. (eds.) *Agonist and Antagonist Actions of Narcotic Analgesic Drugs.* (Proceedings of Symposium of the British Pharmacological Society, Aberdeen, July 1971), (London: Macmillan Press)
Villarreal, J. E. and Karbowski, M. G. (1974). In Braude, M. C., Harris, L. S., May, E. L., Smith, J. P. and Villarreal, J. E. (eds.) *Narcotics Antagonists. Advances in Biochemical Psychopharmacology. Vol. 8* (New York: Raven Press)
Wetli, C. V. and Bednorczyk, L. R. (1980). *S. Afr. Med. J.*, **73**, 1205
Woods, J. H. (1977). In *Minutes of Thirty-Ninth Annual Scientific Meeting, Committee on Problems of Drug Dependence, Inc.*, pp. 420–437
Woods, J. H. (1978). In: *Minutes of Fortieth Annual Scientific Meeting, Committee on Problems of Drug Dependence, Inc.*, p. 658
Woods, J. H., Medzihradsky, F., Smith, C. B., Young, A. M. and Swain, H. H. (1980). *Reported to Forty-Second Scientific Meeting, Committee on Problems of Drug Dependence, Inc.*
Wikler, A., Fraser, H. F. and Isbell, H. (1953). *J. Pharmacol. Exp. Ther.*, **109**, 8

Yanagita, T. (1973). *Bull. Narcot.*, **25 (4)**, 57
Yanagita, T. (1975). *Pharmacol. Rev.*, **27**, 503

5

Cannabis and dependency

Frank Wells

INTRODUCTION

The plant *Cannabis sativa*, from which the psychoactive cannabinols are derived, is related to the nettle, and grows freely in warm climates where it may reach a height of 7.6 m (25 ft). In the United Kingdom it rarely reaches 3 m (10 ft), and may be difficult to germinate. It is, however, a criminal offence in many countries, including the United Kingdom, to grow a cannabis plant, to possess it, or to supply it to others. This fact inevitably means that cannabis derivatives are found in the same environment as other illegal and abused drugs, most of which, in the context of this book, are drugs of dependence. Cannabis, however, is not generally considered as a drug of dependence.

There are many synonyms of cannabis; they include the colloquial 'pot', 'weed', and 'grass', and the preferred American term marijuana, in addition to hemp, hash and hashish. The term 'hashish' is usually reserved for a stronger product, and hash oil is a concentrated extract, highest in active constituents. Ephemeral terms including 'reefer' and 'joint' go in and out of the vocabulary, referring to the physical means whereby the cannabis is used. They are all generic terms which are interpreted differently in various countries, but which all refer to the plant *Cannabis sativa* or less frequently *Cannabis indica* (which is the original indian hemp plant), the leaves, seeds, or other parts thereof, and substances derived therefrom.

The plant is well recognized by its long, palmate leaves, which are saw-edged. The stem, especially beneath the flower heads, is hairy and resinous material is secreted by glands found at the base of these hairs. Cannabis resin, and to a lesser extent the leaves, contains a number of substances, including over 20 different cannabinoids (Madden, 1979); quantitatively the major active component is $\delta 1$ tetrahydrocannabinol, but qualitatively in terms of giving a psychoactive response the most active component is $\delta 9$ tetrahydrocannabinol (THC) (Braude and Szara, 1976). When experimentally administered to human subjects $\delta 9$ THC reproduces the effects of unrefined preparation of cannabis (Isbell *et al.*, 1967), but it is generally considered likely that it is the metabolites of $\delta 9$ THC itself that are most active. (Lemberger *et al.*, 1972). Average cannabis resin has approximately 5% THC content, while cannabis leaf varies from 0.5–2.5% THC content.

HISTORY

It is now recognized that cannabis has been grown since at least the 15th century BC, but its use for 3500 years has always been somewhat paradoxical. It has been said to be an aphrodisiac, or alternatively to repress sexual urge; it is considered an 'energizer' (stimulant) by manual workers in the Caribbean, but they also use it to go to sleep at night. In China, where it was first grown, it was recognized as an intoxicant, amongst other things. It moved across to India and the Middle East, and in its time has been tried in the treatment of virtually every disease. As well as being used as a 'medicinal' drug, it was also used as a 'fashionable' habit especially on the Continent a century ago. Hallucinations were well described by Jacques Moreau in 1845, all attributed to the recreational use of cannabis, which had been well established in social circles (Kalent and Oriana, 1971). Since then, its social use has spread throughout Europe, and its acceptance in America has led to its legal use in some states, notably California. In the United Kingdom its social though illegal use has increased by orders of magnitude since 1945, and it is now estimated that 3 million persons regularly use it.

During the 20th century abuse of drugs in the United Kingdom had never assumed alarming enough proportions to cause concern until the early 1960s although there was a period during and immediately after the First World War when opiates were a temporary problem. In 1916 trafficking in cocaine had assumed 'huge dimensions'; the Defence of the Realm Act was strengthened in 1917, and repealed when the Dangerous Drugs Act 1920 was introduced.

In the years prior to the Second World War the only illicit traffic in drugs recognized as existing in the United Kingdom had been in respect of opium, but in the late 1940s – the immediate postwar years – large-scale immigration from the West Indies and West Africa brought to the United Kingdom for the first time a considerable number of persons used to smoking cannabis. In the early 1950s it became clear that illicit trafficking in cannabis was assuming much greater significance than trafficking in cocaine, opium and other narcotics. At the same time it was apparent that the practice of smoking cannabis had spread to sections of the population who had not used narcotics. Throughout the 1950s the use of cannabis continued to be of real concern only in towns with a large immigrant population, but in the early 1960s it became far more widespread throughout the youth community of the country.

Clearly evidence of this came to light in 1962 when the Metropolitan Police arrested four youngsters in possession of cannabis, and established that there was a well-established traffic in the drug between North Africa and the United Kingdom. During the 1960s cannabis was known to have entered the country from Morocco, Nepal, Afghanistan, Turkey, Israel, Iran, and elsewhere. For the first time cannabis resin was illegally being imported.

Before 1955 few persons were convicted of offences in respect of cannabis; in 1956 there were 103 convictions, 2393 in 1967, and in 1980 over 10 000.

In order to legislate against the use of cannabis, the Dangerous Drugs Act was amended in 1962 to create an offence of permitting premises to be used for smoking or dealing in cannabis, or of being concerned with the management of such premises; these offences had only existed previously in respect of opium, preferred for smoking. The legislation was actually introduced in 1964 and in 1971 the Misuse of Drugs Act was passed.

Cannabis is not prescribed by doctors, but although its use is illegal it has become widespread in certain sections of society. The Misuse of Drugs Act 1971 was passed to give more flexible and comprehensive control over the misuse of drugs of all kinds than was possible under the previous Dangerous Drugs Act. Drugs are put into three classes according to their harmfulness, and the penalties for their misuse are graded accordingly; cannabis is included in class B. Prosecutions since 1971 in connection with cannabis have all been under the Misuse of Drugs Act.

Medical uses for it have been suggested, but therapeutic indications are by no means accepted, even using purified THC, and other more conventional alternatives exist which are more effective for most patients. It would, however, be quite wrong to presume that no medical use for cannabis derivatives will ever be found, and further investigation is entirely justified where there is a possibility that THC or other cannabinoids might become used for valid treatment (Sallan *et al.*, 1980). This point is discussed below.

PHYSIOLOGY

It has long been known that cannabis materials are more potent when smoked than when taken orally, and it has been estimated that there is a threefold increase in potency when the drug is smoked (Isbell and Jasinski, 1969). THC is very lipid-soluble, and it is not surprising that the lipoprotein surfactant lining of the alveoli should prove an excellent vehicle for its absorption. Once it is absorbed through the alveoli, it is rapidly converted to a more active metabolite, but it is a potent substance and as little as 5 mg in a cigarette produces a measurable response (Hochman and Brill, 1971).

Absorption of δ9 THC is almost complete when it is taken orally, but the rate of absorption through the gut is very variable. As THC has high lipid solubility, it is likely that absorption occurs through the upper intestine, and the rate depends on a number of factors including gastrointestinal motility, and the presence of other substances in the digestive tract. Effects are first noticed after about 30 min, and the peak plasma level occurs after about 3 h, then falls during the following 7 h. When smoked, the effects are felt within a few minutes, the peak is up to 30 min later, and the fall off of effects takes approximately 2 h (Lemberger, Axelrod and Kopin, 1971). By either route, plasma concentrations of THC are well related to clinical effects.

The distribution of THC in the body is naturally concentrated and stored in tissue rich in lipid, including the brain; thus plasma concentration falls to a certain level reasonably quickly, but is followed by much slower total elimination of THC or its metabolites due to slow release into the plasma of the substance stored in the fatty tissues. The implications of this are that much higher concentrations of cannabis derivatives than can be detected in the blood are held in significant organs including the brain, and may have variable long-term effects on the organs concerned, possibly accounting for the increasing number of long-term hazards of cannabis use now being recognized, to which reference will be made later. Excretion of THC, and eventually of its metabolites, is in the urine.

BEHAVIOURAL EFFECTS

Tetrahydrocannibol (THC) has a number of different effects, which vary in different individuals. However, when cannabis is used it is the psychological effects that are sought, and these depend to a considerable extent on the dose level, the expectation of the individual, previous experience with the drug, and to a lesser extent on the social environment in which it is being used. A placebo effect has been suggested, and indeed suggestion plays a large part in modifying the effects.

The influence of expectation probably accounts in part for the fact that experienced users of the drug achieve an effect using smaller doses than originally (Jones, 1971). This is the so-called 'reversed tolerance'. There may also be a physiological explanation for this not as yet discovered, but it has already been suggested that enzyme induction, in the conversion of δ9-THC into its more potent metabolites, may develop with increasing use of the drug.

There is an initial period of stimulation, with some anxiety at first, heightened perception, and euphoria, followed by a period of sedation, with a feeling of relaxation and drowsiness. During the first period, usually when in the company of others, the user may be vivacious, chatty, and even garrulous; in the sedative period the user becomes withdrawn, indifferent, and maybe morose.

Overlying both these periods are effects which could be hallucinatory, or psychotomimetic, of which much the most chai istic is altered time perception. Estimations of time are almost ε prolonged, and many studies have confirmed this (Clark, Hough Nakashima, 1970; Weil, Zinberg and Nelson, 1968). Other imp symptoms include impairment of short-term memory and concentration, difficulty in carrying out specific tasks, including driving; conversation may be disjointed, interrupted by gaps in the stream of thought, and reaction time is impaired (Hollister and Gillespie, 1970).

The other psychotomimetic effects include enhancement, either pleasant or unpleasant, of various sensations, such as light, hearing, touch, taste and smell. Also, under the influence of cannabis, art forms, both visual and aural (particularly music) may be more keenly appreciated. However there can occur an unpleasant degree of apprehension about life in general or nothing in particular, or depersonalization, and genuine hallucinations affecting any of the senses (Tart, 1970).

BEHAVIOURAL EFFECTS OF CHRONIC CANNABIS USE

A comprehensive study in the United States (Kolansky and Law, 1971) reviewed the cannabis-smoking habits of a large number of American adolescents; 38 patients from the ages of 13 to 24, all of whom smoked cannabis twice a week or more, were examined over a period of 5 years, and all showed adverse psychological effects. Some also had neurological symptoms. Before using cannabis none of these patients had shown any psychotic symptoms at all, nor had a family history of psychosis, nor had any delinquency been recorded in their family upbringing.

The cases were divided into five groups:

(1) Four patients between 14 and 17 years old had developed a psychotic illness with suicidal attempts.
(2) Four patients between the ages of 18 and 24 had developed psychotic illness without suicidal attempts.
(3) Twelve patients between 15 and 18 years old had developed marked personality changes and were assessed while on trial for possessing cannabis.
(4) Six patients from 14 to 20 years old had developed severe personality changes which at first were not thought to be associated with cannabis use, but which on close questioning were found to be closely related to the onset of heavy use of the drug.
(5) Thirteen young girls aged upwards from 13 years old had marked personality changes with sexual promiscuity; seven of these girls became pregnant, one several times. Sexual promiscuity had not been seen in any of these patients before cannabis smoking.

It was found that some of the parents of these adolescents studied were ambivalent about the effects of cannabis, and had not insisted that the child should not use the drug; the lack of firm guidance was a constant feature in the family and social history of all the adolescents with psychotic symptoms. It appears that cannabis interrupts the normal adolescent growth processes and the youngster concerned may reach chronological adulthood without achieving mental, emotional and affective development.

The long-term effects of chronic cannabis use on the brain and behaviour are considered in more detail below (p. 112–14).

PHYSICAL EFFECTS

Physical effects of cannabis include tachycardia, a rise in blood pressure, redness of the conjunctivae, and dryness of the mouth. Muscle weakness is a regular complaint, and all these physical effects have been measured experimentally (Hollister and Gillespie, 1970). The EEG changes are rather variable in different subjects, but those who have regularly performed EEGs confirm that there is some slowing of rhythm, particularly in the waking EEG, and slightly increased alpha activity. It appears that low doses of cannabis have a sedative effect, but that high doses are stimulating and interfere with the induction of sleep (Tart and Crawford, 1970). This would certainly be compatible with the observed behaviour of regular cannabis users, who, after smoking moderate amounts of the drug, appear content to discuss matters of little consequence long into the night, but the following morning are unable to recall the content of the conversation.

TOLERANCE

Despite anecdotal evidence that tolerance to cannabis might not occur, or that the opposite occurs – that is, reversed tolerance (see p. 106) whereby the experienced user makes do with a less active drug – there is now enough factual evidence to show that tolerance to high-dose levels of cannabis does in fact occur (Hollister, 1979). The demonstration of tolerance in man has inevitably been delayed because of the ethical implications of giving high doses experimentally; but studies have now been done using up to 210 mg/day in divided doses for up to 30 days, which prove that this level of dosage certainly produces tolerance. The relevance of this in society generally is of course debatable, because of the atypically high dose involved. Similar tolerance, however, has been demonstrated in subjects smoking just one cannabis cigarette compulsorily per day, then as desired, which is much more relevant, as it more closely resembles the social pattern of cannabis use (Nowlan and Cohen, 1977). Nevertheless, on the available evidence, the conclusions which can be reached regarding cannabis tolerance are that it is probably not a problem when doses are small or infrequent or when the pattern of use of the drug is not prolonged, but that it does become a major factor when cannabis use is high, sustained, and prolonged. As most social use of the drug does not come into this category, tolerance has not been considered a major issue. Were the pattern of use to change, for whatever reason, the issue might assume much greater significance.

DEPENDENCE

Physical dependence on cannabis or its derivatives is rare, but it can occur. Psychological dependence, while not common, occurs more frequently. International reports have shown that chronic users of cannabis may refuse to stop using it even when it is manifestly obvious to all concerned that their involvement with the drug is adversely affecting their lives, and economic and social status, and is constantly throwing them in conflict with the law (Madden, 1979). Where supplies are in jeopardy, those who are psychologically dependent may become dealers in cannabis to ensure maintenance of their supplies.

The reports of physical dependence on cannabis are worth reviewing, although they are few in number; they indicate that if cannabis were to become a legalized drug, some short-term problems with physical dependence could follow. Withdrawal symptoms were first described in Indian soldiers in the Second World War (Fraser, 1949), and some smokers of hashish in Egypt and elsewhere in the Middle East showed withdrawal symptoms which included sweating, tremors, acute anxiety and depression lasting for 5–7 days (Kielholz and Ladewig, 1970). Two South African reports of similar withdrawal symptoms, lasting up to a week, are worth noting (Bensusan, 1971; Morley, Logie and Bensusan, 1973). It is particularly interesting that from some American states, where a more liberal attitude to cannabis has been adopted, reports are being made of withdrawal symptoms arising in persons who have become very frequent users of the more potent forms of cannabis (Teitel, 1977). Experiments on volunteers have also confirmed that physical dependence does occur when cannabis is administered at short intervals and in very high doses, with mood changes, sweating, nausea, restlessness and disturbed sleep as the most prominent withdrawal symptoms (Jones, Berowitz and Bachman, 1976).

Viewed in perspective, it may be noted that while physical dependence has been described and confirmed it appears to be of short duration, and occurs only rarely, relative to the numbers of persons using cannabis and its derivatives throughout the world. This is a problem which can, therefore, be considered almost non-existent.

There is never any withdrawal syndrome comparable to that produced by suddenly stopping the use of narcotics, alcohol, or barbiturates. However, although there is a relatively insignificant *physical* withdrawal problem, there remains a much greater degree of *psychological* dependence, which is associated with all drugs which have a superficially desirable psychoactive effect.

TOXICITY

If it is presumed for the sake of discussion that there are few known therapeutic uses for cannabis, even for pure δ9-THC, the phenomena observed when it is used could nearly all be called toxic reactions.

Occasionally an acute psychiatric reaction occurs to just one dose of cannabis, in which the subject experiences panic, intense depression, a sense of unreality concerning the environment or even the body itself, paranoid delusions, hallucinations, and delirium. All of this can be aggravated if the user is a novice and is apprehensive about smoking cannabis for the first time. Fortunately, the symptoms subside spontaneously, and only sedation during the psychotic episode needs to be given (Leading article, 1970). Other acute toxic reactions can occur if a large amount of cannabis is smoked at once, leading to cardiovascular shock, with hypertension, tachycardia, and possibly coma. Death has probably been produced by cannabis overdosage (Graham, 1976).

TOXICITY TO THE RESPIRATORY SYSTEM

Chronic cannabis toxicity is most likely to occur in those smoking it regularly in reasonable quantities. It has been repeatedly confirmed that when it is consumed by smoking and the portal of entry of the drug is the lung, cannabis may have several acute and chronic local adverse effects (Henderson, Tennant and Guerry, 1972; Maugh, 1974; Nahas *et al.*, 1974). Repeated smoking of both tobacco and cannabis causes damage to the respiratory mucosa, but that caused by cannabis is greater; admittedly this may be due to the other constituents of cannabis leaf and resin which may be present in the cigarette, but which cannot be separated from the THC component. Nevertheless it is still 'cannabis' that causes it. As a result, there may be a greater incidence of pharyngitis and bronchitis in cannabis users (Braude and Szara, 1976; Taskin, Shapiro and Frank, 1976).

In the alveoli themselves the effect of cannabis, as opposed to that of tobacco, is to impair the natural defence mechanism, which exists to resist pulmonary bacterial infection. There is an in-built antibacterial activity of the alveoli which is significantly impaired by cannabis smoke. The implication of this is that there will be a greater incidence of lung infection, specifically pneumonia, because the natural resistance to bacterial infection has been damaged. There is thus no doubt that cannabis is considerably more directly toxic to the lung than tobacco.

Most members of the public are aware of the relationship between smoking tobacco and lung cancer. It is of interest that much research has been conducted to establish the correlation, if any, between smoking cannabis and lung cancer. The conclusion reached, after carefully comparing the effects of both tobacco and cannabis smoke on human lung and human breast cancer cultures, is that there is a significantly higher frequency of mitotic changes in the cells treated with cannabis smoke (Leuchtenberger, Leuchtenberger, and Chapuis, 1979). This does not allow the conclusion to be drawn that cannabis causes lung cancer more frequently than does tobacco, but it justifies further studies being carried out in known long-term cannabis smokers to see whether there is a greater incidence in the development of lung cancer than either in the

may be extended to humans. In the studies concerned, the THC plasma concentration reached in the animals treated with cannabis, by regular smoking, was similar to that reached in man, thus adding more weight to the justification for extrapolating conclusions in the monkey experiments to humans (Heath *et al.*, 1979).

This particular evidence is important; nearly all cannabis consumption is by smoking, and the long-term effects of equivalent amounts of smoking for periods of 3–6 months produce changes in EEG recordings that are not found in monkeys which have smoked placebo substances for the same period of time. When the monkeys with these abnormal EEGs are killed, and brain tissue is removed, synapses in the limbic system examined under the electron microscope are damaged, which may account for the abnormal EEG and most significantly for the abnormal behaviour associated with it. The abnormalities occur with no other known drugs, and behaviourally include impaired memory and concentration, and emotional instability.

Other changes confirmed experimentally include biochemical disturbances in the brains of newborn animals of various species, whose mothers had been treated with THC (Nahas, 1979). It could obviously be argued that biochemical changes in the brain of a newborn mouse whose mother had received intravenous THC during pregnancy has nothing whatever to do with the function of the brain of a newborn human whose mother had smoked cannabis during early pregnancy. Nevertheless, the abnormal biochemistry reported in animals is associated with abnormal behaviour, and is found in all species in which experiments have been carried out. It cannot be presumed, therefore, that *no* changes will be produced in man which may be permanent, especially when abnormalities of brain function in man are well documented and well recognized.

Apart from animal studies, there are many reports of persistent behavioural abnormalities in human subjects who have been regular users of cannabis (Beaubrun and Knight, 1973; Campbell *et al.*, 1971; Chopra, 1971; Paton and Pertwee, 1973). These are all difficult to assess for a variety of reasons, and most of these reports have been challenged; frequently the users have been shown to include a large number of persons with pre-existing psychological abnormalities anyway, so it has been difficult not to conclude that these pre-existing psychological abnormalities have not predisposed to subsequent cannabis use. This, however, must be an erroneous argument, as a large number of cannabis users certainly do not show any personality or psychiatric defect before starting to use cannabis regularly, but have only subsequently developed significant behavioural abnormalities. The most recent experimental studies continue to confirm that normal animals, assessed by as many parameters as possible, when subjected to chronic cannabis use do develop significant behavioural changes (Nahas, 1979).

Reports from countries where cannabis has been socially available for centuries have suggested that it causes loss of initiative and drive – the so-called 'amotivational syndrome'. It is alleged that heavy long-term use can lead to a state of chronic lassitude with lack of ambition, indifference to the environment, and a 'dropout' way of life (Milner, 1977; Sharma, 1975). It is difficult to be quite certain that these reports do not merely reflect the way of life adopted by some regular cannabis users in the countries concerned as a matter of deliberate choice. There is, however, strong though not conclusive evidence that a chronic state of diminished motivation and social disruption may be induced by regular cannabis use (Edwards, 1976).

Chronic psychosis is a disease well known to be exceedingly difficult to treat successfully. The schizophrenic patient may remain unstable throughout life despite the responsible use of modern therapy. The question arises whether cannabis can induce a chronic psychotic state which remains permanent, demanding constant treatment. There are a number of reports of a persisting schizophrenic-like illness which develops in long-term users of the drug, but it is difficult to exclude other factors which may predominate in the causation of such an illness. Chief of these is the probability of a predisposition to a schizophrenic state, or even latent schizophrenia which is unmasked by the use of cannabis (Leading article, 1976). Nevertheless the data is already sufficient to suggest that long-term consumption of cannabis might lead to the manifestation of a schizophrenic psychosis, whether it was pre-existing or not, and that in itself is an important fact in assessing the validity of its use within society.

A specific review of patients with a history of prolonged cannabis use confirms the eventual development of psychosis, but in some users a degree of tolerance develops as expected until apparently a saturation point is reached which is rapidly followed by the development of a psychosis (Thacone and Shukla, 1976).

Another study conducted in India involved the review of 2000 patients attending a psychiatric clinic, of whom 8.5% admitted regular cannabis use; but it must be remembered that although there is a strong subculture of cannabis use in India, by contrast in some religious sects there is strict abstinence from it. There appeared to be a strong connection between the use of cannabis, and the development of certain types of mental illness, either the unmasking of a latent psychosis, or the aggravation of pre-existing psychiatric disease (Bagadia *et al.*, 1975).

The clinical significance of cannabis in the development of schizophrenia and other psychoses, despite these positive reports, still remains controversial. However, very few psychiatrists would disagree with the rule that no patient suffering from confirmed schizophrenic-type illness should ever use cannabis; the very nature of the diagnosis means that this rule will frequently be broken by the patients themselves, but the concept is still valid (Treffert, 1978).

THE EFFECT OF CANNABIS ON PAIN THRESHOLD, AND ON MEMORY

There is some evidence that regular high levels of cannabis use enhances pain (Hill *et al.*, 1974) but studies of cannabis on the pain threshold are somewhat inconsistent. Nevertheless, a recent study has suggested that cannabis does indeed enhance the perception of pain (Clark *et al.*, 1979). This study also refers to the impairment of memory which occurs in long-term cannabis users. The persons concerned were studied in a carefully controlled environment and had no access to any drugs other than cannabis; they were found to have significant impairment of recall or retrieval memory whether they were moderate or heavy users of cannabis. The heavy users – that is smoking up to 14 cigarettes per day – were found to suffer from a memory storage defect as well. Thus heavy cannabis smokers may find that not only can they not recall events which occurred in the past, but they may not have retained evidence of the event at all.

THERAPEUTIC USES

Although it has been available as an unrefined plant material for decades, and as purified δ9-THC for at least a decade, the therapeutic uses of cannabis remain strictly limited and it is not licensed for use in any form in the United Kingdom. This does not, however, inhibit approved research into possible uses. Research has shown that THC has some place in the reduction of intraocular pressure in acute glaucoma, but in controlled clinical trials it has not proved to be any more effective than pilocarpine, and in fact is much more prone to side-effects. It has also been used in the control of nausea and vomiting produced by cancer chemotherapeutic agents, but again it has proved no more effective than phenothiazines or other conventional antiemetics in the majority of patients. The pharmaceutical industry has conducted research into derivatives of THC, and has produced a number of related cannabinoids; one of these, nabilone, was extensively tested in the United States, and found to be significantly more effective than THC in reducing intraocular pressure, and relieving nausea. It was also found to be free from apparent side-effects. Clinical trials, however, were stopped because of the degree of toxicity discovered in animal studies (Nahas, 1979).

Other derivatives of THC have been investigated, as have other cannabinoids derived from cannabis itself. One of these is cannabidiol (CBD), which is not a psychoactive drug. It has been found to have a potent anticonvulsant effect in rats, and that effect has also been confirmed in humans. What is most interesting is that THC has just the opposite effect, actually triggering certain forms of epilepsy (Karler, Cely and Turkanis, 1973). This fact justifies advising any patient with epilepsy not to use or experiment with cannabis.

SAFETY AND EFFICACY

When considering cannabis, the user takes it because of the effect it has on the brain; for the same reason, doctors give psychotropic drugs of known quality and effectiveness to patients whose medical condition requires them. The doctors, however, are treating patients, not normal subjects, and they are aware of the toxicity of the drugs they are using, so they will use them for as long as necessary, weighing their safety against efficiency. Cannabis does not have a medical use in this context, and its safety must be considered much more carefully if it is to be classed as an effective substance which should freely be available to all who wish for it. It would not appear to fulfil the safety criteria in very many respects.

REFERENCES

Bagadia, V. N. *et al.* (1975). In *Proceedings of the 31st International Conference on Alcoholism and Drug Dependence*, pp. 454–461. (Lausanne: International Council on Alcoholism and Addictions)

Beaubrun, M. and Knight, F. (1973). *Am. J. Psychiatry*, **130**, 309

Bensusan, A. D. (1971). *Br. Med. J.*, **2**, 112

Braude, M. and Szara, S. (eds.) (1976). *The Pharmacology of Marijuana*. (New York: Raven Press)

Campbell, A. M. G. *et al.*, (1971). *Lancet*, **2**, 1219

Carchman, R. A., End, D. W. and Parker, M. R. (1979). In *Rheims Symposium*. pp. 219–227. (London: Pergamon Press)

Chopra, S. G. (1971). *Bull. Narcot.*, **23**, 15

Clark, L. D., Houglas, R. and Nakashima, F. N. (1970). *Arch. Gen. Psychiatry*, **23**, 193

Clark, W. C. *et al.* (1979). In *Rheims Symposium*. 665–680. (London: Pergamon Press)

Cohen, S. (1976). *Ann. NY Acad. Sci.*, **282**, 211

Cozens, D. D., Clark, R. and Palmer, A. K. (1979). In *Rheims Symposium*. pp. 469–477 (London: Pergamon Press)

Dombush, R. L. and Kohodny, R. C. (1978). *Eighth Annual Meeting of the Reproductive Biology Research Foundation, St Louis, 5–9 November*

Edwards, G. (1976). *Cannabis and Health*. pp. 321–342 (London: Academic Press)

Fraser, J. D. (1949). *Lancet*, **2**, 747

Graham, J. D. P. (1976). *Cannabis and Health*, pp. 271–320. (London: Academic Press)

Heath, R. G. *et al.* (1979). In *Rheims Symposium*. pp. 713–730. (London: Pergamon Press)

Hembrea, W. C., Nahas, G. G., Zeidenberg, P. and Huang, H. F. S. (1979). In *Rheims Symposium*. pp. 429–439. (London: Pergamon Press)

Henderson, R. L., Tennant, F. S. and Guerry, R. (1979). *Arch. Otolaryngol.*, **95**, 248

Hill, S. Y. *et al.* (1974). *J. Pharmacol. Exp. Ther.*, **180**, 415

Hochman, J. S. and Brill, N. Q. (1971). *Dis. Nerv. Syst.*, **32**, 676

Hollister, L. E. (1979). In *Rheims Symposium*. pp. 585–589. (London: Pergamon Press)

Hollister, L. E. and Gillespie, H. E. (1970). *Arch. Gen. Psychiatry*, **23**, 199

Isbell, H. *et al.* (1967). *Psychopharmacologia*, **11**, 184

Isbell, H., Jasinski, J. (1969). *Psychopharmacologia*, **14**, 115

Jones, R. T. (1971). *Pharmacol. Rev.*, **23**, 368

Jones, R. T., Berowitz, N. and Bachman, J. (1976). *Ann. NY Acad. Sci.*, **282**, 221

Kalant, H. and Oriana, J. (1971). *Int. J. Addict.*, **6**, 553

Karler, R., Cely, W. and Turkanis, S. A. (1973). *Life Sci.*, **13**, 1527

Kielholz, R. and Ladewig, G. (1970). *German Med. J.*, **95**, 101

Kolansky, H. and Law, W. T. (1971). *J. Am. Med. Assoc.*, **216(3)**, 486

Leading article (1970). *Lancet*, **2**, 1350

Leading article (1976). *Br. Med. J.*, **2**, 1092
Lemberger, L., Axelrod, J. and Kopin, I. J. (1971). *Pharmacol. Rev.*, **23**, 371
Lemberger, J. *et al.* (1972). *N. Eng. J. Med.*, **286**, 685
Leuchtenberger, C., Leuchtenberger, R. and Chapius, L. (1979). In *Rheims Symposium*. pp. 209–217. (London: Pergamon Press)
Madden, J. S. (1979). *Alchohol and Drug Dependence*, pp. 176–184. (Bristol: John Wright)
Maugh, T. H. (1974). *Science*, **184**, 683
Milner, G. (1977). *Aust. Fam. Physic.*, **6**, 1370
Morley, J. E., Logie, P. and Bensusan, A. D. (1973). *S. Afr. Med. J.*, **47**, 1145
Nahas, G. G. (1979). *J. Am. Med. Assoc.*, **242**, 2775
Nahas, G. G. *et al.* (1974). *Science*, **183**, 419
Nowlan, R. and Cohen, S. (1977). *Clin. Pharmacol. Ther.*, **22**, 550
Paton, W. D. M. and Pertwee, R. G. (1973). In R. Melchoulam. *Marijuana*. (New York: Academic Press)
Rosencrantz, R., Fleischman, R. W., and Baker, J. R. (1978). *17th Annual Meeting of the Society of Toxicology* (abstract), **158**, 139
Sallan, S. E., Cronin, C., Zelen, M. and Zinberg, N. E. (1980). *N. Engl. J. Med.*, **295**, 135
Sharma, B. P. (1975). *Br. J. Psychiatry*, **127**, 550
Stefanis, C. N. and Issidoricles, M. R. (1976). In G. G. Nahas (ed.). *Marijuana; Chemistry, Biochemistry and Cellular Effects*, pp. 533–550. (New York: Springer-Verlag)
Tart, C. T. (1970). *Nature* (London), **226**, 701
Tart, C. T. and Crawford, H. J. (1970). *Psychophysiology*, **7**, 348
Tashkin, D. P., Shapiro, B. J. and Frank, I. M. (1976). In S. C. Braude and S. Szara (eds.), *Pharmacology of Marijuana*, pp. 785–801. (New York: Raven Press)
Teitel, B. (1977). *Am. J. Psychiatry*, **134**, 587
Tennant, F. S. and Groesbeck, C. J. (1972). *Arch. Gen. Psychiatry.*, **27**, 133
Thacone, V. R. and Shukla, S. R. P. (1976). *Arch. Gen. Psychiatry*, **33**, 383
Treffert, D. A. (1978). *Am. J. Psychiatry*, **135**, 1213
Weil, A. T., Zinberg, N. E. and Nelson, J. M. (1968). *Science*, **162**, 1234

6

Alcohol dependence: The 'lack of control' over alcohol and its implications

(Can alcoholics become safe moderate drinkers?)

M. M. Glatt

Alcohol and other drugs, as well as alcoholism and other forms of drug dependence, have always been emotionally highly charged subjects – as reflected in the furious controversies in the past between the 'dry' (those against alcohol) and the 'wet' (those for alcohol), and among the 'dry' between the (legal) suppressionists and the (moral) persuasionists (Glatt, 1958); and as regards other drugs, in the 'battle of the barbiturates' (in the 1920s and 1930s) (Glatt, 1962), and in more recent years in the heated arguments between those for and against legalization of cannabis. With regard to alcoholism at the present time, a recent article in the *British Medical Journal* says that 'one particular issue that has generated much heat is whether controlled drinking rather than abstinence is an acceptable aim of treatment' (Smith, 1981); more commonly the argument is seen as one between those who (like Alcoholics Anonymous) believe that in alcoholics only total abstinence from alcohol can lead to a state of happy functioning and a satisfied way of living ('contented sobriety'), and others who feel that a minority of alcoholics (at least) can learn to drink in a controlled manner and live happily that way.

DEFINITIONS

Before trying to enter into the discussion of the latter questions we first have to try and define what in this context is meant by the terms 'alcoholics' and 'moderate' or 'controlled drinkers'. There have been many definitions of the terms 'alcoholism' and '*alcoholics*'. Our own definition (Glatt, 1982) (resembling the one put forward by Davies, 1973) would be: 'Alcoholics are those individuals whose continual or frequent heavy drinking has led to psychological and/or physical dependence and/or physical/psychological/social damage'.

There is of course a definite correlation between alcohol dependence and alcohol-induced damage but it is possible to be alcohol-dependent without suffering damage or complications, and vice versa (Glatt, 1974, 1982). The main part of our discussion will deal with the question of the possibility of controlled drinking in those drinkers who have become dependent upon alcohol (Jellinek's (1960) 'gamma' and 'delta' alcoholics); thus a few words may perhaps not be out of place about the question of moderate drinking in those alcoholics who, without being dependent upon alcohol, have nonetheless developed definite physical or mental complications (as may happen in Jellinek's 'beta' type of alcoholic). As such drinkers do not suffer from 'loss (or lack) of control' (see below), and thus do not have to resist a strong desire to continue drinking once they have started it on a given occasion, there would theoretically perhaps be no reason in their case against moderate drinking. On the other hand, one does not know at present what effect further, even moderate, drinking might have on tissues that have already shown their susceptibility or vulnerability to alcohol. In fact, specialist physicians have often advised, or stressed the necessity for, abstinence in drinkers suffering from chronic pancreatitis, hepatitis, porphyria and liver cirrhosis (Rosch, 1974); alcoholic cardiomyopathy (Annaes, 1974); and seizures (Wessely, 1973). As regards the liver, Davis (1980) has recently expressed the view that moderate drinking might be possible in the case of fatty liver but not cirrhotic liver.

Abstinence has recently also been found helpful in the case of minor brain damage caused by heavy drinking, with improvement in psychological performance and a slower and less striking improvement in the CT scan appearances (Bergman, 1980; Leading article, 1981; Lishman, 1980, 1981). The question has indeed been raised whether 'minor brain damage [could] play a part in precipitating loss of control of drinking . . . [and] explain the poor judgment and repeated relapse into drinking shown by so many alcoholics?' (Leading article, 1981). As CT scanning has demonstrated brain changes in heavy drinkers much earlier and more frequently than previously thought, such questions become even more significant. The possible harmful effect of continued, even moderate, drinking on tissues already alcohol-damaged should not be ignored in discussions on the relative merits and risks of abstinence or controlled drinking approaches in alcoholics (Annaes, 1974; Bergman *et al.*, 1980; Davis, 1980; Glatt, 1976, 1982; Jellinek, 1960; Leading article, 1981; Lishman, 1981; Lishman *et al.*, 1980; Rosch, 1974; Wessely *et al.*, 1973). According to a very recent editorial in the *British Medical Journal* (Portal, 1981) 'the . . . clinician (should) advise abstinence at the first indication of disturbed cardiac function, when the damage may yet be repaired'.

As for 'moderate' or 'controlled' drinking, the terminology, as so often in alcohol-related problems, is in a state of hopeless confusion. Terms such as these and also 'normal', 'disciplined', 'social', 'harm-free' or 'problem-free' are often used interchangeably without any attempt at a definition (Arroyave and McKeown, 1981; Heather and Robertson, 1981). Of course what may be 'normal' drinking for one individual may be too much for another of a lesser weight, or a different sex, or older in age; there are differences and variations in tolerance to alcohol between individuals and in the same individual at different times (Arroyave and McKeown, 1981; Glatt, 1965). Many alcoholics report that in later stages of their disorder they are affected by much smaller amounts of alcohol than in the past (Glatt, 1961, p. 88).

Arroyave and McKeown (1981) defined 'controlled drinking' as 'the drinking of self-monitored amounts of alcohol in nonclinical settings to an extent that does not interfere with functioning in any area (intellectual, affective, physical, legal, or social) and retaining the ability to stop at will or whenever external circumstances render it appropriate'. As to the term 'controlled drinking', strictly speaking if certain drinkers feel a need to control their drinking and to be on guard much or most of the time – unlike the pleasurable, relaxed 'normal', drinking of the ordinary, social drinker – this is unlikely to be satisfying and may indicate a persistent pathological preoccupation with alcohol (Glatt, 1979, 1980). In the words of Chalmers (1979):

> In controlled drinking alcohol is still the central focus of the alcoholic's life, and this is one of its pathological features. . . . The difference between the alcoholic's and the non-alcoholic's drinking seems basically to be that the alcoholic recognises the need to keep his drinking under control for, if he does not, disaster follows. The non-alcoholic sees no need to keep a check on himself.

Moreover, 'normal' drinking might presumably also include the possibility of rarely or occasionally getting 'high', 'merry' or quite intoxicated. While cases have been described of this happening without further 'craving' or mishaps to alcoholics who usually drink in a 'controlled' way, one wonders what the family of such a 'controlled' alcoholic drinker might feel under these circumstances; their old fears and grim forebodings might easily be rekindled with possible repercussions on their attitude to the alcoholic and in turn to the latter's peace of mind and reactions. At any rate, all the terms used (social, moderate, normal, etc.) are imprecise, and in order to avoid repetitions of the same term, with the exception of 'normal', they will be used interchangeably in the following text.

Dependence is another term requiring definition here. 'Drug dependence' (of which alcoholism is one example) was defined by a WHO Expert Committee (1964) as '. . . a state arising from repeated administration of a drug on a periodic or continuous basis'. 'Physical dependence' is 'an adaptive state of physiological change in the body' which manifests itself by the development of (possibly quite severe) physical disturbances if the drug (in our case alcohol) is suddenly withdrawn or its dose markedly reduced very rapidly. 'Psychological dependence' has been defined as 'a state of mind or psychic drive which requires periodic or chronic administration of the drug for pleasure or discomfort' (WHO, 1964).

THE 'TRADITIONAL' OR 'CONVENTIONAL' MODEL OF ALCOHOLISM

Paradoxically, what was known not so long ago (from the 1930s to the 1960s) as the modern scientific approach to alcoholism – has now been dubbed in some quarters the 'traditional' or 'conventional' approach (Pattison, Sobell and Sobell, 1977). It goes back to the scientific work and writings of E. M. Jellinek and the practical achievements of Alcoholics Anonymous, both originating in the mid-1930s. This approach was based on the disease concept of alcoholism with its underlying hypothesis of the 'loss of control' over alcohol (Jellinek, 1960) – and arising from it, the demand for total abstinence. Jellinek (1952b) regarded the loss of control as 'a disease condition *per se*' superimposed on psychological pathology. The loss of control hypothesis seems fundamental to the disease concept of alcoholism and to the question of whether alcoholics can become safe moderate drinkers.

A critical discussion of certain 'traditional concept propositions' was presented by three prominent adherents of 'revised models' and 'alternative approaches' (in the main, 'controlled drinking') – Pattison, Sobell and Sobell (1977) – in their interesting and valuable book *Emerging Concepts of Alcohol Dependence*. Their description of the 'traditional' concepts of alcoholism is based mainly on three sources of reference which they regard as representative: the published literature of Alcoholics Anonymous, Jellinek's publications, and various 'influential' interpretations of the work of Jellinek and Alcoholics Anonymous written by other prominent people (such as Marty Mann, 1968). Some 'propositions' are of interest for our later discussions, among them 'proposition 2': 'Alcoholics and prealcoholics are essentially different from non-alcoholics'. In this context the authors – discussing the suggestion of pre-existing physical abnormality (that is, prior to the onset of alcoholism) – quote a statement by Gitlow (1968): 'This may or may not be so but many people believe that such a (prealcoholic) biochemical defect does exist'. 'Proposition 3' is: 'Alcoholics may sometimes experience an irresistible physical craving for alcohol, or a strong psychological compulsion to drink'; 'proposition 4': 'Alcoholics gradually develop a process called "loss of control" over drinking, and possibly even an inability to stop drinking'. In Jellinek's view loss of control 'was presumed to have a physiological basis and indicated that a person was physically dependent on alcohol'. Pattison, Sobell and Sobell (1977) comment that 'there are at least two major ways of defining loss of control – one (such as Jellinek and Alcoholics Anonymous) centering on physical reactions to alcohol, and the other focusing on volitional behaviour'. According to 'proposition 5': 'Alcoholism is a permanent and irreversible condition'. Pattison, Sobell and Sobell (1977) believe that there are three underlying basic premises for this notion:

(1) a possible biogenetic defect;
(2) the possibility of permanent physiological change resulting from chronic ingestion of alcohol;
(3) 'the belief, which is most represented in traditional notions, that alcoholics are never able to drink again, appears to be due to clinical experience of alcoholics and those in the helping professions who have known or worked with alcoholics.'

Pattison, Sobell and Sobell (1977), however, add the comment that 'traditional approaches except those which postulate pre-existing biochemical defects in alcoholics...could easily incorporate a proposition of reversibility – that biological changes which result from excessive use of alcohol are largely acute in nature and disappear over time', like other reversible disease processes.

CRITICISMS OF THE ABSTINENCE-ORIENTED ('TRADITIONAL') APPROACHES

In recent years the abstinence-oriented approaches have come under fire from various quarters (mainly sociologists, behavioural psychologists, and some psychiatrists), and apparently much more so in Great Britain than in the United States and elsewhere. For example, in France and Germany – both countries with considerable alcoholism rates – controlled drinking is practically 'no issue' (as the present writer has been told by various French and German authorities). It is interesting, for example, that when the question of 'alternative approaches' to the treatment of alcoholism – that is, controlled drinking – is discussed by the leader writers in the *British Medical Journal* and *Lancet*, the American work usually mentioned is that by Pattison, the Sobells and the Rand Reports (Armor, Polich and Stamboul, 1976, 1978) all on the whole in favour of controlled drinking – whereas the views to the contrary held by the great majority of American clinicians are usually completely ignored.

The attacks on the abstinence-oriented approaches have arisen for a variety of reasons: (1) follow-up studies; (2) experimental studies; (3) controlled drinking programmes.

FOLLOW-UP STUDIES

A number of follow-up studies of abstinence-oriented programmes have reported that a certain proportion of alcoholics have become moderate drinkers, for example, 5.8% out of a total of 3847 alcoholics in a number of investigations reviewed by Emrick (1974). Although not the first to find cases of moderate drinking among alcoholics, it was Davies' (1962) report of 'normal drinking' by seven out of 93 former alcoholic patients (who had been drinking uneventfully for between 7 and 11 years after leaving hospital) that aroused interest and a bitter controversy. Obviously there are great difficulties in obtaining reliable follow-up results, particularly in the case of alcoholics, even when complemented by inquiries from collateral sources, such as the family. This difficulty, encountered by every worker in this field, is well demonstrated in the case of Davies' (1962) study. In spite of all his endeavours to obtain a reliable follow-up, it turned out years later 'that one of his ex-patients reported as having...returned to normal drinking had in fact been drinking very heavily all the time'. When during the follow-up the Maudsley research worker had come for an independent interview with the ex-patient's wife, 'the alcoholic patient let his wife know in advance that "he'd bash the living daylights out of her if she told the truth" about his drinking, and she gave an account which was entirely false to substantiate his own false account' (Davies, 1979). This is not mentioned here in order to criticize Davies' study but it clearly illustrates the notorious problems arising in such follow-up studies with alcoholic patients and the caution needed in drawing definite conclusions from them. At any rate, many cases of controlled drinking by alcoholics similar to those reported by Davies have been described in the literature (a few before him and many more since), which has been well summarized by Pattison, Sobell and Sobell and by Heather and Robertson (1981). It hardly needs mentioning that certain other follow-ups came to quite different conclusions, such as those carried out by Pittman and Tate (1972) who did not find any 'normal social drinking' among 255 alcoholics.

EXPERIMENTAL STUDIES

A number of experimental studies have shown that small amounts of alcoholic drink do not necessarily lead to immediate 'loss of control' and drunkenness. For example, Merry (1966) found no difference in the strength of craving between those hospitalized alcoholics who (unbeknown to them) were given vodka and others who received a placebo; Engle and Williams' (1972) study showed that the psychological factor of merely informing alcoholics that there was alcohol in the drink had a greater effect on their desire to drink than the actual presence of alcohol in the beverage; and Mello and Mendelson (1972) found that in a situation where they had unlimited access to alcohol, alcoholics did not even finish all the drink available to them.

CONTROLLED DRINKING PROGRAMMES

A number of therapists reported success in controlled drinking programmes aimed at assisting alcoholics to become moderate drinkers. Summarizing 17 such studies, Pattison *et al.* (1977) concluded that '... taken in concert [these studies] provide strong preliminary data that some alcoholics treated in behavioural programmes can learn to drink in a non-problem fashion'; and Heather and Robertson (1981) concluded in regard to 'controlled drinking treatments for clinic alcoholics' that 'Many seriously dependent alcoholics respond to certain controlled drinking treatments by successfully controlling their drinking. The most effective treatments used so far appear to be problem-solving skills training, regulated drinking practice and self-management training.'

Obviously in Heather and Robertson's view not all controlled drinking treatments were reported by the research therapists to have been successful. The bulk of this work has been undertaken in the United States; but in one of the relatively few investigations in this field carried out in Europe, the Viennese workers Czypionka and Demel (1976) reported that their controlled drinking treatments had failed. They regarded a successful result as one in which a patient never exceeded a blood alcohol level of 60 mg/100 ml and only one of their 20 patients achieved this goal. Interestingly, four patients remained abstinent. The strict definition of these authors raises the question as to what constitutes 'success' in controlled drinking programmes which will be discussed below relative to Ewing and Rouse's (1973, 1976) studies. More recently, Marx (1981) reported a 'controlled drinking' study in the same Vienna clinic aimed at an intensive investigation of a few patients. Out of five patients two proved non-starters because their claim of being controlled drinkers in reality meant what the author calls '*kontrolliertes Betrinken*' (controlled intoxication); a third patient, a delta alcoholic, drank in a controlled manner for 6 months but then developed and died from cancer; the two other patients who are continuing in the ongoing study remain 'socially stable' but there is occasional 'loss of control with unintended intoxication ('*Rausch*') and very great difficulties to get back to abstinence and to maintain it in the following days. . . . A return to an unproblematic . . . way of drinking, as that existing before these patients had become dependent, had clearly not been achieved.' Marx (1981) makes the interesting point that 'the desired modified way of drinking requires a large expense in effort on behalf of therapist as well as patients which can be justified only by a research programme'.

Notable among those unsuccessful with a controlled treatment programme are Ewing and Rouse (1973, 1976), who after an initial promising start (1973) and being hopeful* of the feasibility of such a programme ultimately (1976) experienced a 'complete failure' of their study which had started in 1970.

Describing what at the time was 'the longest follow-up study reported . . . of any attempt to train alcoholics to control their drinking' (27–55

*The present author was present during the 1972 International Alcoholism Conference in Amsterdam at a session chaired by Professor Ewing at which researchers actively involved in controlled drinking studies were discussing their findings. Ewing himself was cautious about the ultimate result of his own ongoing investigation which he felt at the time showed promise. The present author – then Editor of the *British Journal of Addiction* – asked Ewing to let the *Journal* have the report of the outcome independent of whether it would turn out to be positive or negative. Ewing agreed and the paper appeared in the British *Journal of Addiction* 4 years later (Ewing and Rouse, 1976).

months after completion of treatment), 35 patients were referred or self-referred to this experimental (outpatient) programme. Of these 14 attended at least six times and nine of them came on 12 to 24 occasions. There was a treatment session each week, lasting at least 4 hours. Ewing and Rouse concluded that 'Although patients who persisted in the programme were very successful in learning to recognize their levels of blood alcohol and at developing controlled drinking patterns while in the programme, the follow-up results indicate that sooner or later all of them had begun to drink again with loss of control'. This happened although:

> All patients who completed the full programme of 12 weekly visits were convinced [at that time] that they had re-established control over their drinking . . . [and] that they had now relegated alcohol to a realistic place in their life pattern and could keep it from again domineering them . . . [In all cases] . . . sooner or later these hopes were dashed. Not all patients required hospitalization for their drinking and not all patients necessarily showed such lengthy, or as many, episodes of loss of control as . . . before the treatment programme. However, for the alcoholic, even one bout of loss of control can be damaging in many ways and, we believe, represents a poor outcome of therapy.

The above statement of these authors' personal view is interesting because it may help to explain the often diametrically opposed conclusions drawn by different observers from their studies as to the successful achievement of 'controlled drinking'. After all, many alcoholics treated by abstinence-oriented programmes also relapse, although a high proportion of these are often reported to be greatly 'improved' in their drinking habits and their general adjustment in life (Clare, 1977; Glatt, 1955, 1959, 1961, p. 183; Royal College of Psychiatrists, 1979). Those who believe in the justification of controlled drinking programmes often argue that '. . . the episodes of loss of control in . . . would-be controlled drinkers represent no more than the relapse of the abstinent alcoholic'. Rejecting this argument, Ewing and Rouse (1976) say 'that if [this were] so, we might expect our patients to be willing to attempt to return to controlled drinking patterns again and again. Instead our patients have spontaneously and voluntarily decided, in the majority of cases, that they must be totally abstinent. . . .'

As described in our own studies below (p. 129), patients failing to achieve controlled drinking on the first attempt often wanted to try again and again, in this way differing from the alcoholics observed by Ewing and Rouse in their much more systematized and planned study. However, the spouses of our patients usually became more and more desperate about these repeated failures (as they saw it) urging us to motivate their alcoholic partner, who often claimed good 'control', to quit drinking for good. Such experiences were usually quite different from the cases of our ex-patients advised to remain abstinent who had occasional relapses into uncontrolled drinking, but whose subjective feelings and statements that they were nevertheless (on the whole) improved were often spontaneously confirmed by their spouses. There may be much less scope for bitter controversy between patient and family as to whether he or she has achieved abstinence than whether he has succeeded in controlling his or her drinking, as the term and the meaning of 'control' lend themselves to various subjective interpretations. However, there must remain a substantial element of subjectivity whether under such circumstances a therapist would regard programmes aiming at either abstinence or 'control' as a success or a failure – the more so as very reliable follow-ups are difficult to carry out, and as even 'collaterals', such as the spouse, cannot always be relied upon to make truthful statements in respect to the partner's maintained improvement or otherwise. Clearly believers in the controlled drinking approach as a practical alternative to abstinence-oriented programmes would not share the view of Ewing and Rouse (1976) that '... even one bout of loss of control ... represents a poor outcome of therapy'. Like Ewing and Rouse, the present author too has often found that '... even one bout of loss of control can be damaging in many ways', in particular to the morale of the alcoholic's family. However, in abstinence programmes – with those patients who show some motivation – such relapses often become progressively rarer and less intense; and their families witnessing this begin to appreciate it and tend to cooperate with treatment and to develop a constructive attitude towards the alcoholic.

On the other hand, those of our alcoholic patients who attempted to control their drinking often seemed to have considerable arguments with their families as to whether they were successful or not. A common initial happening was this: one such outpatient presented himself proudly proclaiming that he was drinking moderately, keeping to the agreed small amounts (see below). His wife, though agreeing that he was 'trying', was convinced that he was drinking much more 'though of course I cannot be sure. After all, he is out of the house all day and I only see him in the evening; from his attitude, his behaviour, his looks, etc. I suspect he has taken some drinks during the day – but he strongly denies this and is getting angry when I question him about it.' In our experience, this is a very typical statement under such circumstances and highlights some of the problems confronting therapists in determining 'outcome' of treatment and in comparing results of abstinence-oriented and controlled drinking programmes. The individual therapist's own emotional bias (obviously based on such experiences) is therefore likely to be an important factor in coming to his decision whether he prefers to encourage abstinence or 'controlled' drinking. 'Based on [their own] experiences with [their] patients and a long-term follow-up', Ewing and Rouse concluded that, 'in [their] hands at least, further attempts to inculcate controlled drinking by such methods are unjustified'. It is interesting that – in spite of so many research reports coming out in favour of controlled drinking over the past two decades – the great majority of clinicians involved in the treatment of alcoholics still aim at abstinence and strongly disagree with statements coming in the main from research workers and 'armchair' reviewers that '... controlled drinking has come to be an accepted aim of treatment ...'. There is, however, a place and indeed a need for such planned programmes to be carried out for research purposes in certain centres. Through such research we can learn more about loss of control and its implications, and the stage and the circumstances where it becomes inadvisable for a 'problem drinker' to continue with controlled drinking because dependence has already started to develop.

JELLINEK'S 'LOSS OF CONTROL' HYPOTHESIS

In view of findings such as those discussed on p. 122 Jellinek's loss of control hypothesis has been seriously criticized, and rejected by some. To a certain extent some criticisms of Jellinek's loss of control hypothesis stem from semantic misunderstandings of his formulation. Loss of control does of course *not* mean – as often misunderstood – that a gamma alcoholic's first drink inevitably and on every occasion necessitates further drinking; what it does mean – as first noted by Jellinek's friend and close colleague Mark Keller (1958) and stressed by the present author on numerous occasions since 1965 (Glatt, 1965, 1966, 1970, 1974, 1975, 1976, 1980, 1982) – is that such a drinker can never be certain that he will be able to call a halt on any given occasion once he has imbibed one or two drinks. This misunderstanding has arisen partly perhaps because Jellinek's first and better known version (Jellinek, 1952a in the WHO Expert Committee Report) described the loss of control as meaning that 'as soon as a small quantity of alcohol enters the organism, a demand for more alcohol is set up .... This demand lasts until the drinker is too intoxicated or too sick to ingest more alcohol.'

Jellinek – as Keller (1972) related – immediately realized his error committed in the haste of going to press and in the same year published a corrected version (Jellinek, 1952b), saying that 'Any drinking of alcohol starts a chain reaction which is felt by the drinker as a physical demand for alcohol. This state ... may take hours or weeks for its full development.' Obviously Jellinek knew fully well – as Keller explains and as every clinician working regularly with alcoholics knows – that many alcoholics do not necessarily *always* have to continue after having had a drink or two. In his book *The Disease Concept of Alcoholism* Jellinek (1960) mentioned that a very perplexing characteristic of the loss of control phenomenon was that 'loss of control does not emerge suddenly but rather progressively and that it does not occur inevitably as often as the gamma alcoholic (i.e. the loss of control type of alcoholic) takes a drink'. There seems therefore little point in carrying out – as has been done repeatedly – complicated tests in hospital that prove that alcoholics do not always have to go on drinking after the first glass. Such experiences by no means prove that the loss of control hypothesis is a 'myth'. What all these findings imply, however, is that the notion of loss of control as a permanent irreversible organic phenomenon seems untenable with the possible exception referred to above (p. 123) of types of alcoholism that may have arisen on the basis of a pre-existing biochemical defect (Pattison, Sobell and Sobell, 1977) (or where such defects may have developed secondarily during the course of heavy drinking).

AUTHORS' INVESTIGATIONS

PATIENTS' RETROSPECTIVE REPORTS

As regards our own experience, a certain proportion of our alcoholic patients have always maintained that before presenting themselves in the clinic, they had been able (occasionally or in other cases quite frequently) to stop their drinking on a given occasion after a few drinks (Glatt, 1976). Since first reporting on these investigations at an international meeting in Oslo in 1965 (Glatt, 1967), I have taken special care in interviewing all my alcoholic patients (amounting to several thousand) at some length about their experiences in this respect, apart from discussing the subject in numerous group therapy sessions with alcoholics. In this way the earlier impressions reported in 1965 could be continually checked and rechecked, and on the whole the patterns reported earlier have been confirmed by the experiences of the much larger numbers of alcoholics interviewed and observed in the intervening 15 years. Thus over the years there emerged certain patterns of circumstances (see below) in which such patients had temporarily managed to achieve short periods of controlled or moderate drinking before ultimately ending up with episodes of uncontrolled drinking.

THE 'GENTLEMAN'S AGREEMENT'

In view of these experiences, since 1962–63 I have adopted a method of 'gentleman's agreement' (Glatt, 1972, 1973) with recently seen alcoholic patients who made it clear from the outset that under no circumstances would they be prepared to undergo treatment aimed at total abstinence without first having been given a fair chance to prove that they could – in spite of their own previous experiences to the contrary – still become moderate drinkers. In order to forestall criticisms that the therapist had strongly influenced the outcome by his own attitude (for example, by precipitating the patient's reaction of uncontrolled drinking as a self-fulfilling prophecy (*Lancet*, 1975) because it was expected by the therapist) such patients were told that there had indeed been a number of reliable reports of alcoholics who managed to revert to 'normal' drinking. The patient was asked to fix a daily low maximum of alcoholic drinks; no matter what the circumstances, he was on no account to drink more than this amount – seeing that the object of the exercise was to prove that he was always in control of the situation and the drink. The amounts finally agreed upon varied but were generally much less than the patient initially suggested; they were usually in the region of up to two to four half-pints or two to four single glasses of spirits or two to four glasses of wine: all these drinks were not to be taken in one session but spaced out over the day.

The patient was also advised about the circumstances that some of our patients in the past had found favourable to their usually very short-lived, maintenance of moderate drinking (see p. 129) – not to drink alone or in company of drinking cronies but rather with moderate drinkers or with the spouse, to drink slowly, preferably with a meal, and not to drink when tense, worried, fatigued, etc. Whenever possible, the patient's spouse was kept in the picture. As a rule, while the alcoholic was quite enthusiastic, spouses were usually highly sceptical and often openly hostile to such arrangements – even though the drinkers had agreed that if the 'gentleman's agreement' should fail, they would accept such failure as evidence that they were not in control of their alcohol consumption (rather vice versa) and that they would then adopt the only possible alternative, that is to abstain totally.

Over the past two decades this approach was adopted by over 300 alcoholics. For technical reasons these were usually private patients, mostly emotionally fairly stable and highly educated men in their 40s or 50s. They were often in high executive or equivalent positions (a few doctors and other professional men were included), usually with a history of considerable professional achievement and success. They still enjoyed the benefits of a stabilizing job and marriage; however, though the latter was still intact, the wives had usually shown growing concern over their husbands' drinking. Their degree of dependence often appeared considerable, as reflected for example in their previous often repeated failure to keep their drinking under control, in spite of their intellectual knowledge of the risks involved in excessive drinking. On the other hand, there were the balancing factors of above-average intelligence and relative emotional and social stability, as reflected in their ability to keep both their highly responsible jobs and the affection of their families, in spite of heavy drinking and its resulting complications. They were, in general, fairly sober when presenting themselves at the first interview, and expressed extreme confidence in their ability to succeed.

However, though theoretically such patients seemed to constitute a relatively promising sample as regards the possibility of controlled drinking, the great majority had not kept to the agreement by the time of the next visit a few weeks later; a few had stuck to it somewhat longer, for weeks or (rarely) months (as far as could be ascertained; see the strictures made above). However, of those alcoholics about whose fate and behaviour we had fairly reliable information (i.e. the great majority), virtually everyone by the end of a year had failed; nevertheless they often remained convinced that they could still learn to drink in moderation, and that it was only unforeseen circumstances that were responsible for their relapses into uncontrolled drinking (such as nagging by the wife, mother-in-law's visit, etc.), so in spite of their families' entreaties, they requested a continuation of the 'gentleman's agreement'.

Such observations confirm, of course, that in many alcoholics the first drink does not immediately trigger off a bout, but also that it is likely to do so sooner or later – as a rule sooner rather than later. The AA slogan of the first drink proving 'fatal' or disastrous, would still seem applicable in the great majority, with the addendum of this happening 'sooner or later'. However, under certain circumstances quite a number of our alcoholic patients managed 'controlled drinking' temporarily before relapsing into uncontrolled drinking. Factors influencing such drinkers' ability to control their drinking, in our experience, appear to be associated with the drinkers' personality and environmental circumstances, as well as with the activity of the 'agent' alcohol (such as the concentration and the amount of drink, and the rapidity with which it is consumed). Thus, in both causation of alcoholism and manifestation of the loss of control, all the members of the triad – 'agent', environment, and 'host' – appear dynamically involved with each other. For example, moderate drinking was more likely to be maintained on the following occasions (Glatt, 1965, 1966, 1972, 1973, 1974, 1975, 1982), when the drinker:

(1) Slowly sipped a relatively weak beverage (beer, wine) or one or two glasses of spirits only (influence of the *agent* (pharmacological factors) on loss of control).
(2) Drank in the company of the spouse or of moderate social drinkers only (thus it was very rare to find an alcoholic wife who drank too much in her husband's company); drank immediately before an assignment, appointment, date, etc. which the drinker regarded as very important and worth making a special effort for; had very little money available, though under such circumstances such drinkers often preferred not to start drinking at all (all influence of *environmental factors* on loss of control).
(3) Drank on a full stomach, shortly before or with a meal – [(*a*) physiological aspect]; drank when contented, cheerful, carefree, in a relaxed frame of mind, free from responsibilities and not tired, etc. [(*b*) psychological aspect] (influence of '*host*' or personality on loss of control).

On the other hand, the same individuals tended to *relapse* into uncontrolled drinking when they

(1) Gulped, rather than sipped spirits or quickly downed quite a number of pints (*agent effect*).
(2) Drank alone at home or in the company of heavy drinkers (*environmental effect*).
(3) Drank on an empty stomach, and particularly when depressed, tense, frustrated, resentful, tired, bored, etc. (*physiological and psychological aspects of the host effect*).

Patients themselves were often aware of some of these risks. In our experience the most important factor in triggering relapses was the drinker's mood or frame of mind at the time of drinking. Not infrequently many patients when asked whether they believed they could drink in moderation replied: 'It depends'; and when asked to be more specific, they often mentioned 'my state of mind at the time of drinking'. Another factor frequently mentioned was the type of drink: 'I'm all right as long as I stick to beer; spirits are my downfall'. Naturally, there is usually an interplay of various factors and there are some individual variations. Some drinkers, for example, stated that they tended to relapse only, or mainly, when in the company of heavy drinkers (being encouraged by their example), but not when drinking at home, even when alone. On the whole, however, the frequent tendency of many alcoholics under certain circumstances to behave in the way depicted above (first described by Glatt, 1965, 1966) was so marked that patients' replies could often be anticipated. The above findings clearly did not imply definite, fixed rules but seemed to depend on the meaning of the total situation for the individual (Glatt, 1973).

However there are usually so many factors involved in the individual case that one can speak only of certain tendencies and not of certainties. Heather and Robertson (1981) in a recent comment and criticism of the present author's '... revision ... (of) the traditional concept of loss of control ...' (Glatt, 1976), write:

> ... Glatt conceded that the 'hypothesis of an irreversible, metabolic change as the basis of loss of control in all types of alcoholism certainly seems untenable'. Nevertheless, the concept of loss of control is defended on the basis of a multi-dimensional conception of alcoholism involving pharmacological, physiological, psychological and sociocultural factors. Unfortunately, however, Glatt... although he mentions several social and psychological 'factors' which may prevent [loss of control] from emerging, fails to address the task of specifying under what conditions it *will* be produced....

Clearly in spite of general tendencies so many interacting factors are involved in activating the 'loss of control' phenomenon in alcoholics that no-one at present can say under what conditions it will definitely be activated; likewise adherents of controlled drinking approaches (such as Heather and Robertson, 1981) cannot be certain under what conditions loss of control can be avoided. What appears probable, however, is that the greater the drinker's degree of dependence, the 'stronger' the effect of the 'agent' (such as 'gulping' a large number of strong drinks) and the more unfavourable the emotional, social and physiological factors (a lonely individual in a state of tension and depression, drinking alone at home on a weekend on an empty stomach), the greater the likelihood of uncontrolled drinking (see p. 131) – although even under such unfavourable circumstances not every alcoholic will always necessarily end up drunk.

From the experiences of a great many of our alcoholic patients it almost seems that many alcoholics might be able to drink more or less moderately as long as they do not really need the drink. On the other hand when they really 'needed' it – for example, looking for the pharmacological effects of alcohol in order to find relief from tension or depression – they either immediately or within a short time became unable to control their drinking. It might thus seem that, paradoxically, alcoholics could more readily 'get away' with moderate drinking as long as they did not really care whether they had a drink, but hardly ever when they really strongly desired or experienced a 'craving' for a drink.

When our alcoholic patients described their relapse after a period of abstinence, more often than not the first drink did not immediately lead to uncontrolled drinking. More commonly what happened was:

> I was curious whether after having had no drink for 3 months I could have a few drinks. So I had a pint, and nothing happened. As I did not feel any craving to have another one, I felt safe and took three pints 2 days later. Again nothing happened, but after a week I had started on a few whiskies, and after 3 weeks I was back to my former drinking pattern and I could not stop.

Another interesting point was the spontaneous statement by quite a few alcoholics that they could stop drinking on a given occasion as long as they did not 'feel' the effects. Depending on other circumstances to some extent, some patients maintained that they were usually able to stop after three, but 'never' after five or six beers; others could fairly safely take two but 'never' four gins. In many others the amount they felt they could take on a given occasion depended on psychological and/or social conditions.

Another interesting observation was that many loss of control alcoholics were able to interrupt their drinking session long before they were '. . . too intoxicated or too sick to ingest more alcohol' as Jellinek's first (1952a) but later corrected (1952b) version of the loss of control principle had defined it. Although in such cases further drink was readily available, such drinkers when closely questioned about those events, usually stated that they had drunk 'enough' – in other words that they had arrived at the 'state' which they had wanted to reach, at least for the time being. Such drinkers sometimes felt a few hours later the need to 'top up', and such drinking occasions which may have started in a loss of control fashion ('gamma') – the first few drinks being immediately followed by further drinking – thus took on the appearance of the 'inability to abstain' ('delta') type within the same bout (see below).

THE CONCEPT OF A 'LOSS OF CONTROL' BLOOD ALCOHOL THRESHOLD-RANGE

In order to account for the frequent finding that some loss of control alcoholics could sometimes stop drinking as long as they did not 'feel' the effect of alcohol, the present author put forward two possible working hypotheses (Glatt, 1965, 1966).

First, the possibility that there may be a varying critical blood alcohol level-range above which the already existing loss of control phenomenon may begin to be activated on a given occasion. The level-range varies from person to person, and in the same individual from time to time, depending on a variety of factors which might be predominantly psychological and/or physiological, psychosomatic, psychopharmacological or psychosocial in nature (Glatt, 1965). The concept of a 'low alcoholic limen', an 'individual alcohol pro mille at which a physical need develops which decides the drinker's further conduct', was put forward by Martensen-Larsen (1950). Within a given drinking occasion, initially – after a drink or two have been taken – psychological and social factors may be relatively more important until the range of 'threshold' level is reached when physiological and pharmacological factors begin their progressively increasing influence. Thus [such an] alcoholic may find it relatively easy to cope with the psychosocial factors after a few drinks, and may experience little craving when taking alcoholic drinks inadvertently, without the intention of changing his 'feeling' state and escaping from stress, and while being treated in a hospital unit.

All these conditions were in existence in Merry's (1966) trial (referred to above, p. 124) in which vodka or a placebo was given surreptitiously to hospitalized alcoholics who under such circumstances with the lower priming dose of 1 fl oz (30 ml) of vodka did not develop any craving. With increasing alcohol concentrations, however, the alcoholic may find it more difficult to tolerate and withstand the pharmacological-biochemical factors that arise from the action of alcohol on the 'host' and may experience a greater craving, as borne out in Merry's (1966) trial, in which craving reactions and scores were found to be much higher when he doubled the surreptitiously given amount of alcohol.

Second, there is the technique of 'disciplined' and rationed drinking so as to remain below the individual 'loss of control' threshold-range (Glatt, 1965).

In Jellinek's (1960) view resumption of drinking in the gamma loss of control alcoholic after a period of sobriety can be ascribed 'not to a compulsion, but rather to an impulse whose danger is not recognized or is explained away'. Loss of control, in Jellinek's view, is characterized by the adaptation of cell metabolism to the presence of alcohol and by acquired increased tissue tolerance. A true physical demand is set up for alcohol which explains the occurrence of withdrawal symptoms during the drinking bout, and these in turn lead to the 'craving' for the expected relief from further drinking. No definite evidence has hitherto been put forward for the existence of a physical demand before the first drink has been taken. Keller (1972) differs from Jellinek on this important point and believes that 'the essential loss of control is that an alcoholic cannot consistently choose whether he shall drink or not . . . and if he drinks, he cannot consistently choose whether he shall stop'. In Keller's view loss of control thus applies also to taking the 'first' drink, the alcoholic having been '. . . compelled to drink by his addictive cue, as if alcohol itself has become such a cue'. This is in clear contrast to Jellinek's view that loss of control only sets in after the first few drinks have been taken. According to Jellinek's hypothesis, even in the gamma alcoholic the take-off into a drinking session may be due to what he has called 'undisciplined drinking', that is '... a deliberate transgression of the social rules relating to amounts, times, occasions and locales of drinking'. Jellinek regarded this type of drinking as characteristic of the 'alpha (symptomatic) alcoholic' who drinks to obtain emotional relief, its importance 'diminish[ing] greatly ...' after loss of control has been established. Reading Jellinek's description of 'undisciplined drinking' and comparing it with the drinking habits of our patients who had temporarily managed moderate drinking, I was struck by the similarity of their technique of avoiding 'undisciplined' drinking by keeping to more or less strict rules regarding 'amounts, times, occasions, locales ...' and spacing out their drinking. Unlike the fully 'practising' alcoholic who rationalizes wildly in order to enable him to go on drinking with a clearer conscience, who is forever 'covering up' for his drinking, and who is not really aware of his impotence *vis-à-vis* alcohol, the type of drinker discussed above was by then quite well aware that he could not really drink like other people. For either (*a*) psychological and/or (*b*) social reasons such drinkers had become aware of the constant need to watch their step in regard to alcohol and to drink warily.

(*a*) *Psychologically* they may have been able to develop a more mature and less impulsive or less 'stupid' attitude towards drinking – no longer or at least not always using alcohol as a means to cope, nor bypassing the necessity of having to cope with internal conflicts and external problems. On the occasions described, such individuals did not start the drinking session with the goal of feeling different. Thus they may have been able to 'discipline' and 'ration' their drinking – without necessarily feeling very content and comfortable – so as to remain well below their threshold level (Glatt, 1965). 'The trouble,' one alcoholic patient told me recently, 'with being advised to discontinue drinking at a certain blood alcohol level in a controlled drinking programme is that it is just then that I feel like going on most strongly.'

(*b*) *Socially* some alcoholics may have benefited by changing their type of job or their environment so that they are no longer exposed either to frustration or resentment, for example, occupational status, domestic relationships etc., or to constant temptation, or to the risks arising from belonging to heavily drinking subgroups and then feeling the social pressure to conform.

Under such psychological or social circumstances some alcoholics who have become aware of the risks of, and the terrible price paid for, heavy drinking somehow manage, usually only temporarily, to discipline their drinking in such a way as to remain below the individual, critical loss of control threshold-range. Conceivably, addicts who are emotionally more stable, particularly after a more radical change of their frustrating environmental situation (occupational, domestic, housing), with a resulting improvement in outlook, hope, and general attitude, might be more capable of this difficult exercise in self-discipline, but even such people will probably find sooner or later that the effort is too great, and then break down again. It may become progressively more difficult for the drinker to withstand the lure to continue drinking on a given occasion, the more he moves into the range of his individual threshold blood levels. This may be because below these levels psychological and psychosocial factors are relatively more important and easier to resist, whereas on the drinking occasions when his threshold-range has been reached, the additional contribution of pharmacological and physiological factors becomes more and more important, these factors are more difficult to tolerate and resist by psychological efforts, such as the drinker's good intentions not to continue drinking.

Such strictly rationed drinking, with the necessity of constantly watching one's step, can hardly be pleasant and satisfying in the long run – and, as stressed by Kjolstad (1963), this technique of 'nibbling' or 'taking nips' can hardly be called 'normal drinking'.

In subsequent years the concept of the individual threshold-range for alcoholics was favourably commented on by some authorities (Arroyave and McKeown 1981; Ewing, 1973; Gross, 1973), but criticized by others (Heather and Robertson, 1981; Paredes *et al.*, 1977). In fact, Heather and Robertson (1981) comment that '... the postulation of such a threshold might be made to account for the negative results of some priming dose experiments', such as that of Merry (1966) and possibly of Hodgson *et al.* (1979) from which '... it might be concluded...that a high dose of alcohol is needed to stimulate craving and subsequent loss of control over drinking behaviour, and that this was the reason why previous experiments have failed to demonstrate it – the priming doses used were too small'. Heather and Robertson (1981), however, regard this as an 'erroneous conclusion ...', seeing that 'Hodgson *et al.* (1979) ... do not claim that the presence of craving in severely dependent alcoholics would always eventuate in uncontrolled drinking ... there is plenty of evidence that even large quantities of alcohol do not necessarily trigger alcohol-seeking behaviour in alcoholics' (Cohen *et al.*, 1977; Gottheil *et al.*, 1972; Mello and Mendelson, 1972; Paredes *et al.*, 1977). Yet in answer to this criticism our threshold concept surely nowhere indicated that higher blood alcohol concentrations always and necessarily activate loss of control behaviour but merely that they are increasingly likely to do so, but always depending on the interaction with psychosocial and other circumstances. There seems to be no conflict in this between our formulation of the threshold concept and the conclusion drawn by Heather and Robertson (1981) from 'the evidence of the Mendelson, Cohen and Gottheil research teams that alcohol addicts who have reached very high blood alcohol levels are able *under appropriate circumstances* [my italics] to moderate their drinking or abstain altogether'.

The criticism by Paredes *et al.* (1977) of our threshold concept is also based on the demonstration by various studies that '... persons who have been repeatedly addicted to alcohol can consume enough alcohol to obtain a blood alcohol concentration of 140 mg/100 ml on two consecutive days without developing physical dependence....These and similar findings seriously challenge [Glatt's] notion of a critical blood alcohol concentration threshold for *initiating* physical dependence' [my italics]. However my threshold concept was not – as stated by Paredes *et al.* – the suggestion that loss of control would not be 'initiated' until a critical blood alcohol concentration threshold had been exceeded, but merely that in an individual with already established loss of control, reaching or exceeding the threshold-range might under certain circumstances activate the loss of control phenomenon. It does not imply that it would definitely cause it, in the first place, by reaching such levels on a few isolated occasions. In fact, I would tend to agree with Paredes *et al.* (1977) when they continue: 'It may well be the case that physical dependence is initiated by drinking over a sufficient length of time *and* maintaining a sufficiently high blood alcohol concentration'. In this connection they point to studies such as Mendelson (1964) which demonstrated experimentally that 'continuous sufficient drinking does initiate a physical dependence process followed by a withdrawal syndrome . . .'.

An interesting rebuttal of the criticism referred to above (Heather and Robertson, 1981; Paredes *et al.*, 1977) that the repeated finding that even high blood alcohol levels did not necessarily trigger off loss of control spoke against the threshold concept, was voiced by the late M. M. Gross (1973), a well-known experienced clinician who in this context stressed his involvement with alcoholics in a research-laboratory setting. He pointed out that

> . . . people in laboratory experiments with self-regulated drinking administration who are alleged not to have shown any loss of control, because they did not drink every drop that they could have drunk, nevertheless drank enormous quantities of alcohol. That point is overlooked in the critiques from the self-administration experience. It is said that someone might have had 30 ounces, but he only drank 28, so that therefore was no loss of control! I wonder how many normals would drink 28 ounces, even apart from the issue of tolerance – the reaction to the drink? . . . . A further contingency is that in addition to . . . Glatt's remarks about the threshold beyond which there is apparently a loss of control – a lower threshold – . . . there is probably [also] an upper threshold, in terms of critical levels of alcohol continuing over a period, when they get so sick that they stop. In other words there is something that initiates it at the bottom end, and something that turns it off at the top, which . . . helps better to explain phenomenologically what is going on.

It would therefore seem that the threshold-range concept developed on the basis of our clinical experiences with alcoholic patients is on the whole consistent with experimental findings and not invalidated by findings in studies demonstrating that alcoholics could stop drinking even in the presence of very high blood alcohol levels.

RELATIVE 'LACK OF CONTROL' RATHER THAN ABSOLUTE 'LOSS OF CONTROL'

Observations made by our patients over many years confirm that in many loss of control alcoholics the first drink, or even the first two or three, do not necessarily precipitate a drinking bout – at least not immediately. Indeed, it might seem more correct to state that the first drink in the great majority of alcoholics leads to a drinking bout *sooner or later* but not usually on the very first occasion. The exception perhaps is in those in later stages of the disorder and with severe degrees of dependence, and even then this is not always the case. Nonetheless there is undoubted value in AA slogans such as 'one drink, one drunk' or 'the first drink is fatal' in indicating to alcoholics the enormous risks involved in having *any* alcoholic drink. It is surely much easier to resist temptation before there is any alcohol in the bloodstream, rather than adding its significant pharmacological effect on the organism to the psychological and social factors which probably triggered the heavy drinking in the first place. But alcoholics should also clearly be made aware of the fact that while they should try to keep off the first drink, all is not inevitably lost if they have tasted it, for example, accidentally. They cannot, and should not, argue 'as I am doomed anyway I can just as well continue drinking'. Even after a few drinks the 'host' can often assert itself and withstand the increasing desire to continue drinking.

At any rate the majority of our alcohol-dependent individuals seemed to exhibit not a *static and absolute* loss of control but rather a *relative and variable* lack of control. This is a progressive phenomenon in many but by no means all alcoholics who continue drinking. It occurs, as stated by many patients, with increasing frequency in later stages of alcoholism (Glatt, 1973), and apparently also when a larger amount of alcohol or more concentrated alcoholic drinks are taken. From statements made by many hundreds of our alcoholic patients, and many of their close relatives, it would seem that the lack of control phenomenon – a concept resembling or overlapping with Edwards *et al.*'s (1977) 'impaired control over the drug ethyl alcohol' (the leading symptom of their 'alcohol dependence syndrome') – is influenced not only by the activity of the 'agent' alcohol and its effect on the individual's mental and physical state, but also on factors connected with the drinker's personality ('host') and the environment in dynamic interaction with each other. If one abandons the attempts to restrict the meaning of loss of control to biochemical or pharmacological factors, and widens the term to include also the role of psychosomatic and psychosocial factors, many observations in the present study as well as those in the literature, which otherwise seem difficult to explain or harmonize (Heather and Robertson, 1981; Pattison, Sobell and Sobell, 1977), make sense fairly easily.

Personality and environmental factors, as well as the pharmacological action of alcohol itself and any biochemical changes that may have arisen out of interaction between host and agent, as well as other organic alterations (such as early minor cerebral alterations demonstrated by CT scanning (Bergman *et al.*, 1980; Leading article, 1981; Lishman, 1980; Lishman *et al.*, 1980) may influence the working or the activation of the loss of control phenomenon. It is quite likely that this will occur to a different extent in different individuals and even in the same individual at different times under different psychosocial conditions. It would seem that, given some insight, a degree of emotional maturity, considerably altered domestic, occupational, economic and similar circumstances, considerable effort (and perhaps luck) but often even without all this, sometimes even without treatment, some alcoholics are able to manage to stick to relatively small amounts of drink for certain (usually) shortlived periods. Theoretically, it might indeed seem possible for controlled drinking to continue for very long periods (described in the literature) as long as 'the going remains good'. However, many changes affecting personality, environment and agent have to come about and, what is more difficult, to remain if controlled drinking is to continue safely; and with the insecure constellation of 'host' and environmental factors threatened by so many unpredictable internal or external cues or signals which might trigger off a bout, it is unlikely that such dramatic changes will occur very frequently and be maintained for long. As with the average, non-alcoholic person, business will not always continue to be good, the boss may once more make unreasonable demands, the wife may start nagging once again; and the balance between the opposing influences – the 'pull' of the lack of control on the one hand, and the psychosocial factors acting as 'brakes' on the other – may once more be tipped towards a defeat of the controlling or disciplining factors. The ubiquity of unpredictable threatening cues and the likelihood that so many required favourable psychosocial circumstances will not persist for ever, may help to explain why the estimated range for normal drinking among samples of alcoholics reported in the literature by adherents of controlled drinking approaches (Heather and Robertson, 1981; Pattison, 1976), has remained relatively low, between 5 and 15. It may also explain why many experienced clinicians the world over hardly ever encountered clear-cut examples of alcoholics who have achieved safe controlled drinking over lengthy periods. But the frequently made point that if a drinker succeeds in drinking in a controlled way it proves that he has never been an 'alcoholic' in the first place, is a circular argument. One surely cannot strongly advise a drinker, whom one diagnoses an alcoholic, to abstain from drinking, and tell him later when proved wrong that the original diagnosis had been incorrect. However in view of the belief among some adherents of controlled drinking approaches that 'the most immediate and important question . . . in relation to the choice of treatment goal is. . .the client's wishes, beliefs and attitudes about this' (Heather and Robertson, 1981), even those strongly in favour of an abstinence programme might occasionally think it preferable to give a patient who strongly insists that he could drink moderately, the chance to prove it during a preliminary period, as in our 'gentleman's agreement' (see above). As long as he succeeds in this no harm has been done; should he fail, however, he could not afterwards complain, or (more importantly) feel aggrieved, that he has not been given a chance to do it his way. He would then be less resentful and more cooperative with any subsequent abstinence-oriented approach.

Our hypothesis of the multidimensional relative 'lack of control' is clearly different from Jellinek's (1960) 'working hypothesis' of a purely physiopathological basis for 'loss of control'. Jellinek regarded loss of control and pharmacological addiction as synonymous even though, as pointed out by Pattison, Sobell and Sobell (1977), the notion of irreversibility is not a particularly necessary element in the approaches of Jellinek and other 'traditionalists'. In our own hypothesis of social and psychological as well as physiopathological factors being involved in the 'lack of control', the phenomenon in theory could be reversible, though in practice its establishment has indicated a certain vulnerability or susceptibility in the individual drinker which easily might make for 'reinstatement' (Edwards and Gross, 1976) after even a short period of resumed drinking. Reversibility, even in theory, would be impossible in the type of alcoholism caused by pre-existent biogenetic defects though the existence of genetic types of alcoholism is still regarded as doubtful despite the fact that certain recent studies have come out strongly in favour (Goodwin, 1976; Schuckitt *et al.*, 1972). Theoretically reversibility might be less unlikely where physiopathological changes acquired during the course of prolonged drinking may have led to the loss of control and its activation; and least unlikely where psychological or social causes led to excessive drinking and indirectly to loss of control which in such cases may itself also be more subject to psychosocial influences. However, in practice, because of the superimposed multifactorial 'lack of control' an attempted return to 'controlled drinking' seems a very hazardous undertaking in all such types of alcoholism. Jellinek (1960) preferred to talk of the alcoholisms rather than of alcoholism. Indeed the often diametrically opposed findings of so many reputable and reliable research workers in the field of alcoholism are difficult to reconcile with each other unless they deal with different subgroups; and possibly the existence of various overlapping (Davies, 1979) types of alcoholism (Glatt, 1982; Jellinek, 1960) of somewhat different aetiology and with types of loss of control of varying intensity, possible reversibility and prognosis might help to explain some of the problems involved in the loss of control phenomenon.

The WHO Expert Committee on Alcoholism (1965) made a clear distinction between psychological and physical dependence, although not everyone is in agreement with this (Keller, 1980). The possible importance of psychological factors in the loss of control phenomenon, as in our hypothesis, even in the absence of physical factors, is clearly illustrated by the following WHO Expert Committee (1965) definition:

> Drug dependence is a state of psychic or physical dependence, or both on a drug. . . . All these drugs have one effect in common: they are capable of creating, in certain individuals, a particular state of mind that is termed 'psychic dependence' . . . this mental state may be the only factor involved, even in the case of the most intense craving and perpetuation of compulsive abuse . . . psychic dependence can and does develop . . . without any evidence of physical dependence. . . .

Quoting this definition, Pattison, Sobell and Sobell (1977) make the pertinent comment that 'The notion of alcohol addiction [dependence] can connote a pattern of drinking associated with either a state of mind (psychological) or physical withdrawal symptoms or both. Thus a particular pattern of alcohol use may or may not have a physiologic basis.'

Returning to the studies cited above that are usually quoted by those against an exclusive abstinence approach and in favour of an alternative, controlled drinking approach (Heather and Robertson, 1981; Pattison, Sobell and Sobell, 1977), these included follow-up studies that showed a certain proportion of alcoholics had become controlled drinkers; experimental studies showing that small amounts of alcohol do not inevitably and immediately cause loss of control and drunkenness; and therapists reporting successes using behavioural techniques to assist certain alcoholics to become controlled drinkers.

In theory, in view of the theoretical considerations discussed above, and in the light of the multidimensional, relative 'lack of control' hypothesis, such findings reported in the literature in a minority of alcoholic patients studied are understandable without too much difficulty. One interesting finding in this connection – not yet touched upon in our discussion – is the reduction of alcohol consumption sometimes observed in elderly alcoholics (Glatt, 1972, 1978; Murphree, 1976; Williamson, 1978). Such findings appear to illustrate well some of the points discussed above. 'With advancing age, changing psychological, physiological, and socio-economic conditions may affect the balance and dynamic interaction between . . . personality, environment, and the pharmacological effect of alcohol on personality' (Glatt, 1972). Relevant psychosocial factors in this context which affect elderly drinkers include on the one hand, retirement with its loss of status, friends and interest which might make for heavier drinking, but, on the other hand, reduction in financial resources and opportunities for drinking coupled with progressive restriction of physical capacity and mobility which may all severely limit the elderly person's consumption of alcohol. Such psychosocial factors may thus affect the loss of control in elderly alcoholics (Glatt, 1972; Murphree, 1976) in opposite directions.

Those who consider that controlled drinking is an appropriate goal for some alcoholics have attempted to set up tentative guidelines for selection of patients and have considered in this context factors such as the client's wishes and beliefs; attitudes about controlled drinking; the severity of drinking symptoms; age, employment, pretreatment levels of alcohol consumption, etc. (Heather and Robertson, 1981). It has been said that 'both from the theoretical and empirical point of view . . . controlled drinking appears to be an acceptable goal for the early problem drinker, or moderately dependent alcoholic . . . [and that it] is a more likely outcome for the moderately dependent alcoholic than it is for the severely dependent' (Hodgson *et al.*, 1980). But at this juncture an attempted forecast of whether an individual alcohol-dependent patient is likely or not to succeed in this direction is little more than inspired guesswork. In the great majority of cases many years elapse during the drinker's slow, insidious progress from social drinking via relief drinking to 'compulsive' drinking and alcohol dependence, (Glatt, 1961, 1982) and the transitional period between non-dependent and dependent drinking with gradually developing 'lack of control' and with intermediate 'shades of grey' may often be quite lengthy. Obviously there must be a very lengthy period of time during the earlier (Jellinek's (1952b) prealcoholic and prodromal) phases of non-dependent 'problem drinking' when future alcoholics could heed the warning signs and take stock. At least a certain proportion among them may at this stage revert to moderate drinking. It stands to reason that the earlier the 'problem drinker' reaches this point in his downward progress the greater the possibility. Non-psychopathic drinkers who misuse alcohol in the absence of psychological or chemical dependence – that is, by 'choice' rather than 'need' (though there must be a large grey area in between) – or because of socioenvironmental influences – such as drinking haunts, friends and peer-groups, domestic or occupational stress, etc. – should, theoretically, have a relatively fair chance to become safe moderate drinkers. Careful assessment of the stage at which the problem drinker presents himself, of the psychosocial factors contributing to his excessive drinking, the extent to which they could be modified, and the presence and degree of psychological and physical dependence, is therefore very important. It appears likely that in the drinking population at large there must be many relatively early 'problem drinkers' who are not yet dependent and who could become moderate drinkers. However, among the problem drinkers who come to the attention of helping agencies, clinics etc., those who are already clearly dependent probably form a very high proportion. As a rule it is those very drinkers with a long history of severe alcohol misuse and clear evidence of dependence who, because of this strong dependence, are most vociferous in claiming that in spite of all their previous failures they could still drink 'normally'.

The concept of a relative 'lack of control' in place of an absolute 'loss of control' readily explains why a certain proportion of our alcoholic patients managed – though rather uneasily and insecurely – occasional episodes of usually shortlived 'controlled drinking'. In most of these patients over the years loss of control occurred more and more frequently but only in a minority did loss of control become 'overwhelming' in the sense that it occurred on practically every drinking occasion. As we have seen in many patients, certain psychosocial circumstances and factors felt by the drinker to be sufficiently significant could act as a brake and help him temporarily resist the urge to continue drinking. Other factors of possible importance in the activation of the 'loss of control' may be: drinking on an empty stomach which helps the drinker to 'feel' the effect of alcohol more quickly (one of the obvious reasons why alcoholics as a rule prefer to drink without eating at the time), a decrease of alcohol tolerance in the relatively late phases of the drinking career (Glatt, 1982); and, usually earlier than this, liver changes and brain atrophy demonstrated by CT-scan appearances

(Bergman *et al.*, 1980; Leading article, 1981; Lishman, 1981; Lishman *et al.*, 1980). Such changes may increase the effect of alcohol on the brain but may also reduce the drinker's ability to resist the pull of the loss of control by impairing the strength of his superego. The fact that such factors – the alcoholic's common neglect of food intake, the fatty liver changes, and (at least to some extent) the brain changes demonstrated by CT scan – are reversible, may contribute to the variability of activation of loss of control in alcoholics. At any rate the influence of psychological and social factors on the drinker's behaviour obviously do not come to an end with the gradual development of the loss of control but persist afterwards, though the pharmacological effect of the 'agent' and its interaction with the host-personality gradually become increasingly important. Among the agent-factors is (as discussed above) the size of the priming dose – this is not identical with the threshold-range concept which is an interactional, multidimensional concept. The effect of the priming dose largely depends on 'host' and environmental factors being involved at the same time – a view in line with that of Hodgson (1980) that the possible priming effect of a few strong drinks '. . . is now considered to be just one component of a multivariate framework'.

Younger age, low severity of drinking problems and regular employment are 'variables [that] have emerged as the strongest predictors of a controlled drinking outcome' (Heather and Robertson, 1981). It is often said that it would be quite unreasonable to expect young alcoholics to accept total abstinence from alcoholic drink, 'reasonable to expect' that young alcoholics 'who have had a drink problem for a shorter period [than the average alcoholic] might be more able to control their drinking' (Oxford and Edwards, 1977). But apart from the duration and the severity of the drink problem ('agent'), personality factors such as emotional maturity, ego-strength, frustration, tolerance, etc. are of great importance in this connection. People who have become dependent on alcohol at a young age are often more immature than their peers – the chances of them growing up emotionally by using difficulties as challenges to be overcome and thereby as spurs to emotional growth are reduced by their drinking. The ability of such young alcoholics to forego immediate gratification of their strong desire to continue drinking on a given occasion just before they begin to feel the effect they anticipate and want, is often much lower than that of older, emotionally more mature alcoholics. In the case of these young alcoholics, therefore, the factors of both 'personality' (and probably often also environment, such as heavily drinking peer-groups and subcultures) and 'agent' cause opposing outcomes of controlled drinking approaches. It has rightly been said that treatment goals should be realistic and tailored to the individual and that it is pointless, even harmful, to attempt to impose limits which the patient will not contemplate, but such limits can be proposed and negotiated' (Anonymous, 1981). Possibly some young alcoholics who accept an abstinence goal for several years, may subsequently, in view of their increased emotional maturity, the relatively shorter duration and lesser severity of their drink problem, stand a better chance of controlled drinking than when first seen. Discussing such possibilities with young alcoholics who initially refuse to cooperate with abstinence-oriented treatment after, and even though, they have previously failed to control their drinking, might help to motivate them to consider at least a temporary abstinence goal.

GAMMA (LOSS OF CONTROL) AND DELTA (INABILITY TO ABSTAIN) ALCOHOLISM

Psychosocial factors, in our view, do not only influence the loss of control phenomenon but also whether the individual drinker on a given occasion presents as a gamma or a delta-type of alcoholic (Glatt, 1972). In Jellinek's (1965) view these types of alcoholism are the only ones which could be regarded as physical 'addictions' and 'diseases, since it is the adaptation of cell metabolism, and acquired increased tissue tolerance and the withdrawal symptoms, which bring about craving and loss of control (gamma) or inability to abstain (delta)'.

Gamma alcoholism is said to be the most common type in predominantly spirit-drinking countries, and the delta type is predominant in France and other wine-drinking countries. The difference between gamma and delta types, according to Jellinek's (1960) 'conjecture' was mainly a matter of the different 'agents':

> . . . the delta alcoholic . . . spreads beverages of low alcohol concentration over some 16 hours of the day – and the total of the drug is a large amount – the cell metabolism [of nervous tissue] is continually conditioned to the presence of alcohol; but in the gamma alcoholic who drinks concentrated spirits in a concentrated period of time, the metabolism of nervous tissue cells becomes conditioned by the 'signal' of the 'first drink'.

However, it is well known that both these types can occur in all countries, and most of our alcoholic patients seen in recent years seem to exhibit both types at different times, often depending on *environmental* circumstances. For example, the alcoholic who starts drinking in the morning and knows he will always have drink available later during this day, may only have a few drinks in the morning and 'top up' intermittently during the rest of the day (delta); but the same man, fearing that he will not be in a position to drink later on, may 'let himself go' and quickly finish half a bottle of whisky or more (gamma). The husband drinking after work in the evening, in the pub knowing that his wife has clearly told him that on no account would he ever be allowed again to drink at home because of his previous drunken behaviour, may 'make hay while the sun shines' and drink as much as he can in the pub (gamma) before staggering home; however, after divorce and a new marriage to a more 'understanding' wife who initially does not object to his drinking at home, the same man may only drink a little of the bottle in the pub and take the rest home, secure in the knowledge that he may be able to finish the rest at leisure at home over the next few hours (delta).

'*Host*' factors too may be important in differentiating gamma and delta drinking behaviour. Individuals with a higher frustration tolerance and a stronger conscience may be able to delay giving in to their craving to have more and more drink for a much longer time – some hours (delta) – and proceed with their work before having more drinks; whereas the man with a much lower frustration tolerance and a lower ability to endure deprivation may have to satisfy his craving immediately after his first few drinks (gamma) independent of work obligations (Glatt, 1972). Our view is in line with Keller's (1972) idea that 'the main difference [between the delta and the gamma type] is in approaching the needed state of intoxication gradually if one has the leisure, or more rapidly if one has to meet in-between responsibilities. Or sometimes . . . some addicts simply lack the opportunity which they may dearly long for, to nibble between bouts, while others have the opportunity.'

Delta alcoholism may be more prevalent in France, not only as Jellinek (1960) believed, because of the predominance of wine-drinking (a weaker agent than the spirits favoured in countries where gamma alcoholism is more prevalent), but also because social factors and habits allow the French drinker to go on nibbling alcohol intermittently all day long without feeling guilty or rejected by his friends and neighbours. Such an activity would be widely frowned upon in Anglo-Saxon countries, where the alcoholic needing a certain amount of alcohol over 24 hours does not have the opportunity to space it out throughout the whole of the day; thus he has to gulp it down quickly, possibly directly from the bottle in a locked bathroom where he imbibes as much as he can in the short time available to him.

If this view is accepted, then gamma and delta alcoholics are not all that different from each other, and both are affected by psychosocial as well as pharmacological and physiological factors.

FAMILY ATTITUDES TO CONTROLLED DRINKING

Alcoholism is a family illness, and when discussing the possibility of a controlled drinking approach with an alcoholic, the attitude of the long-suffering family should not be ignored. The drinker himself may only be too keen or willing to choose the controlled drinking alternative in preference to the abstinence approach. The alcoholic's wife who does not have the 'benefit' of her husband's frequent amnesias for his drunken exploits (which help the alcoholic to continue drinking with a less troubled conscience), and lacks his unbounded optimism, is usually much more pessimistic. She may be forgiven for thinking that she has heard it all before – her husband's numerous, recurring protestations that this time it will be different, that in spite of it all he will prove to her that he can drink in moderation. The spouse's scepticism may further increase the usually already existing bitter family disharmony. Where behavioural approaches are employed it would therefore seem necessary also to try to alter the wife's attitude. This applies particularly to one who has been so conditioned by her husband's frequent failures in the past that she expects him to fail to control his drinking – an attitude which in turn may easily make such an approach much more difficult for her husband (Glatt, 1982).

THEORY AND PRACTICE

Various researchers have reported successes with behavioural approaches aimed at helping alcoholics to become moderate drinkers. In theory, as we have seen above, there may be no reason why the great majority of alcoholics could not achieve such a goal. As they can do it for short periods why should they not be able to keep it up for a lengthier period. In practice, however, most clinicians are confronted daily by alcoholics who have tried controlled drinking in the past and have failed again and again. It is an exception to meet a new alcoholic patient without a history of many failures in such attempts. As regards behavioural approaches, innumerable and often quite unpredictable psychosocial, psychosomatic and other factors may at any time act as internal or external cues that could trigger off relapses, so that even the most conscientious and effort-consuming therapeutic–prophylactic efforts in that direction will find it quite impossible to 'immunize' the drinker against more than a small fraction of such possible risks and contingencies (Glatt, 1976). There is of course also the well-known difference between hospital and laboratory conditions on the one hand, and 'field' situations on the other hand, so that it is often doubtful whether the 'success' reached in hospital will be maintained after the patient has left hospital.

As to the likely success, or otherwise, of behavioural approaches it has been pointed out that there may be a possible fundamental difference between conditions such as phobias – which the patient loathes, badly wants to get rid of, and wants nothing better than for the treatment to succeed fully – and a condition such as alcoholism where very often the patient is at best ambivalent, one half of him fully realizing that he ought to give up drink, and the other fearing and nostalgically regretting the possible loss of subjective, fleeting yet immediate positive 'rewards' from his drinking, should treatment succeed. After all, many alcoholics only enjoy drinking after reaching the blood alcohol levels where they begin to 'feel' the effect.

As regards the possible 'trigger' situations that might spark off a relapse and that might be forestalled by appropriate behavioural or cognitive techniques, one additional problem is that a very common (indeed probably the most common) reason for a relapse is the alcoholic's persistent hope that he can still be a moderate drinker after a period of abstinence. So he may start drinking again in the absence of any clear-cut internal or external cues (Glatt, 1976, 1982). Thus, in addition to behavioural techniques, psychodynamic and psychosocial approaches would seem necessary to try to change underlying attitudes and to induce the missing motivation. Although behavioural techniques have only been mentioned in association with controlled-drinking approaches, they can of course, and have been, used to assist the alcoholic towards abstinence, in association with other methods.

Extensive research in all aspects of lack of control is undoubtedly necessary in order to understand more about the phenomenon that in spite of many criticisms is much more than a 'myth' and appears fundamental to the understanding of alcoholism. Such research, however, should be carried out only at certain centres and by experienced workers belonging to various professional disciplines on interested and selected patients. As yet research results hardly justify holding out to the general population of alcoholics the hope of long, continued, safe controlled drinking. At the present juncture this seems to be within the reach of only relatively few, and probably relatively early-phase, alcoholics, apart from non-dependent 'problem drinkers'. Although the importance of this is doubted by some (Heather and Robertson, 1981), many clinicians in actual practice must have quite frequently come across alcoholics, abstinent for years, who after hearing or reading glowing reports about controlled drinking attempted it, only to end up drunk within a short period*. What might be even more risky is the effect of overconfident pronouncements of the possibility of controlled drinking on the motivation of alcoholics who have not come to the notice of interested agencies but who are encouraged by their suffering relatives to do 'something'. Such alcoholics could go on rationalizing their endless failure to control their drinking by saying: 'well, I will just keep on trying. I know I can, many others have done it.'

*A few hours after these lines were written the writer saw an alcoholic patient and his wife who confirmed his account: 'My husband had been abstinent for 6 months. Both of us were then told by a friend that he had just read in a medical journal that some alcoholics could be controlled drinkers. My husband later that day took a few light beers. He felt fine and continued like that for a week. He then switched to stronger beers for another week. The week after it was whisky, and about a month after his first beer he was back to needing half a bottle of whisky each day as in the past.' Incidentally this type of downward progression after the first few drinks – taking from several days to several weeks between the 'first drink' and the gradual development of uncontrolled drinking – appears much more common than the usual version of the first drink leading to a bout on the same day (Glatt, 1982). This gradual onset of uncontrolled drinking is of course very well known among alcoholics and clearly illustrates the advisability to speak of a relative 'lack' rather than an absolute 'loss' of control over alcohol. There seems little point in disproving by complex hospital and laboratory tests that the first drink induces a craving of such overwhelming intensity that it immediately and inevitably necessitates further drinks until the drinker is intoxicated. Again, most papers coming out strongly in favour of controlled drinking 'prove' their point by disproving a view which Jellinek (1952a) never held and by quoting a statement made in an 'unguarded moment' (Keller, 1972) and corrected by Jellinek (1952b) almost immediately. Instead of impressing uninitiated readers with reams of evidence that the first drink does not trigger off an immediate bout, those in favour of controlled-drinking approaches should perhaps concentrate on demonstrating that a few drinks can be safely taken by alcoholics without the likelihood that in the great majority fairly soon an uncontrolled bout will follow, and on researching whether reliable guidelines can be discovered as to the type of alcoholic individual who stands a good chance of becoming a safe controlled drinker.

Wallace (1979), a strict adherent to the abstinence approach, stated that

> As a programme administrator ... accountable for the lives of a large number of alcoholics, I have no choice but to advocate abstinence, since research to date ... has failed to provide me with reliable answers to the following questions: 1. How many alcoholics can be expected to be able to drink normally? 2. Over what temporal intervals can the behaviour be maintained? 3. What factors serve to differentiate those who cannot do this from those who can? 4. What levels of risk are there in varying operational definitions of 'normal drinking' for various alcoholic populations given particular individual, situational, and societal constraints? 5. Does a valid technology exist for producing normal drinkers out of alcoholism?

Arroyave and McKeown (1981) (clinicians working in Oxford) expressed their concern about the tendency to make unsupported assertions such as that 'controlled drinking is increasingly accepted as a goal for some alcoholics' (see Hodgson *et al.*, 1978). Of interest in this connection may be a statement by Heather and Robertson (1981), two British protagonists of controlled drinking approaches; their own recent survey showed that 'most (British) treatment centres ... now accept the principle of controlled drinking', but at the same time these authors '... regret the tendency to relegate the new methods to a minor and ancillary role in the range of traditional treatment services – as being applicable, for example, to only those with less serious problems'. Clare (1977) concluded that 'those who admit the possibility of a return to a normal pattern of drinking are usually at pains to point out that it is a realistic option for a minority of alcohol-dependent individuals only, and that total abstention is the only solution for the majority ... [although] permanent abstention is adopted by only a small proportion of patients ...'.

Arroyave and McKeown (1981) also make the criticism that

> The concept of abstinence as the only treatment goal is under increasing attack and is being made to appear old-fashioned, punitive, prejudiced, harsh and unsupportive. By contrast treatments advocating controlled drinking appear as warm, humanitarian, progressive, and attractive in that they would remove many of the tensions from the relationship between the alcoholic and helpers .... The aim of controlled drinking is far from proven as a workable alternative.... Its uncritical sponsors may be identifying excessively with their prospective patients and projecting their own unwillingness to consider the necessity of abstinence. Much of the evidence rests ... on results based on consumption data relating to periods of time and not to people.

At present controlled drinking, they believe, should remain a research area 'with very limited influence on the way in which services for the treatment of alcoholics are organized'. Advocates of controlled drinking approaches 'have yet to be able to identify the alcoholics who can be helped by it and to demonstrate that the final outcome is as effective, in terms of quality of life, as existing treatments aimed at abstinence'. The advantages of the new approaches will have to outweigh the disadvantages arising from the lack of benefit to be derived from AA, and there is need for carefully costing the provision of such services based on such a different philosophy with regard to personnel, training needs, etc. 'Until all this is worked out it would seem sensible to avoid creating illusory hopes and weakening the resolve of the many alcoholics currently attempting abstinence or indeed abandoning present treatment aims simply because of a change of fashion' (Arroyave and McKeown, 1981).

In the case of the complex and heterogeneous conditions of the various alcoholisms, with so many factors – psychological, physiological, pharmacological, sociocultural, economic, etc. involved in dynamic interaction with each other – so many fundamental questions are unanswered that there is a vital need for research in all aspects of alcohol misuse and alcoholism. But as Arroyave and McKeown (1981) rightly stress, while welcoming the 'challenging and questioning of traditional, sometimes dogmatic concepts ... essential to progress ...', one should keep in mind '... the danger of exciting research suggestions leading to premature and ill-judged changes in clinical practice'. Just as clinicians should continually check the impressions gained from their observations by keeping in close touch with the findings of planned, controlled research, so those research workers who are greatly in favour of the 'problem, free-drinking' approaches should take notice of the experience of the majority of clinicians in this field throughout the world who (while not denying the occurrence of the phenomenon) nonetheless hardly ever come across 'normally' drinking alcoholics in their practice. Their experiences tend to bear out a statement made by a prominent recovered alcoholic, R. Brinkley Smithers (1976) (founder of the Smithers' Foundation in New York): '... most [alcoholics who later recovered] experimented with controlled drinking many, many times before they finally realized that abstinence was the only solution and now ... live a life of happy sobriety'.

One particular group of alcoholics in whom perhaps one could expect to find instances of safe controlled drinking are the alcoholic doctors; but, for example, of the 200 or so contacts of the British [alcoholic] Doctors' Group the great majority report numerous trials with controlled drinking. But, as a cofounder of the Group (M. G. K., reported 1980): 'As a group we have yet to learn of a single case of a successful return to "controlled drinking"'.

The conclusion drawn by Heather and Robertson (1981) from their recent survey of the field was that 'clearly controlled drinking treatment is here to stay'. Against this should be set the fact that controlled drinking experiments by 'drunkards' must surely have gone on since prehistoric man discovered what alcoholic drink could do for him – and to him. Controlled drinking may be feasible for the problem drinker who is not dependent, but it seems highly unlikely to apply to the clearly dependent 'alcoholic' in view of the enormous risks involved quite apart from the emotional stress on their sorely tested families. As to alcoholics who have achieved abstinence and a state of contented sobriety, few observers would probably disagree with the conclusion reached by Mark Keller (1972) (in whose view the loss of control symptom may sometimes be in prolonged remission): '. . . so long as no one knows what it takes to reactivate the symptom in any individual who is addicted, the advice is. . . . The prudent alcoholic in remission should not put himself on trial.'

Probably the approach by most therapists to the treatment of alcoholics closely conforms to Madden's (1979) statement: 'The goal of controlled drinking . . . is unattainable for the majority of alcoholics, yet knowledge of its possibility for a few can induce many to disastrous attempts to reach it. . . .At the present time many therapists aim for abstinence among their subjects [but] are not surprised when a few become able to drink moderately.'

To conclude with the three questions and issues (for which research is required and recommended) on 'non-abstinence-oriented treatment' formulated by an expert committee established by the United States Institute of Medicine (1980) at the request of the National Institute on Alcohol Abuse and Alcoholism (NIAAA):

(1) What is the expected number of patients who achieve controlled drinking?
(2) Are the risks of using controlled drinking as an accepted treatment goal justified?
(3) What are distinguishing characteristics, if any, of patients who are most likely to benefit from this approach?

Our own views on the central position of the relative lack of control phenomenon and the related questions of 'abstinence or controlled drinking' are based on, or at least heavily coloured by, clinical experiences and extensive discussions over the past few decades with thousands of alcoholics and their families. Our conclusions on the overriding need for abstinence, not as the goal but as the means to a happy, satisfying life, are likewise derived in the main from having come across a great many fully recovered and abstinent alcoholics and happily reunited families, though unfortunately also many failures – but in spite of all our diligent search and hundreds of 'gentleman's agreements' – the *safely* drinking alcoholic has remained a strangely elusive creature.

To try and answer the question in the title of this chapter – Can alcoholics become moderate drinkers? – For shorter or more rarely longer occasions many alcoholics can undoubtedly drink moderately but, as things stand at present, only a small percentage of dependent alcoholics can hope to become safe moderate drinkers over prolonged periods. No one at present can be sure beforehand which alcoholics may turn out to be in that minority. In statements on that issue a clear difference should be made between those non-dependent 'problem drinkers' who suffer from alcohol-related problems other than dependence, and many of whom probably learn to revert to moderate drinking. Unfortunately, however, it is often the severely dependent alcoholic who may pick up ideas for problem drinkers learning to drink in a controlled manner and may be only too anxious to try such 'new' knowledge out on herself or himself – as a rule with disastrous consequences.

CONCLUSION

The frequent need of the dependent alcoholic to continue drinking once he has taken a few drinks is not necessarily derived – as Jellinek (1960) seems to have thought at one time – from 'physiopathological' processes but from a dynamic interaction of multiple factors pertaining to 'host' (personality) and 'environment' as well as to 'agent' (the pharmacological nature of the drug ethyl alcohol). In the great majority of alcoholics there is no absolute loss of control but rather a multifactorial, relative lack of control. As regards the effect of the 'agent', in dependent drinkers an individual critical threshold-range may be involved. There may be a certain range of blood alcohol levels above which lack of control may be activated, a range varying from person to person and in the same individual from time to time. This will depend on a variety of factors which might be predominantly psychological, and/or physiological, psychosomatic or psychosocial in nature. All other factors being equal, a higher priming dose of alcohol is more likely to activate the already existing 'lack of control' phenomenon than a much lower priming dose; since other, emotional, social, etc. factors are never equal at different times, the priming dose, possibly with the exception of very high amounts, depends for its effect on the interaction with 'host' and environmental factors – which can act either as brakes against activation of the lack of control (for example, a conscientious businessman who has to keep an important appointment); or favour its activation (for example, a lonely, depressed woman who starts to drink on her own at home). The lack of control activation is certainly not always – and probably only infrequently–triggered off immediately by the 'first drink'. The 'loss of control' hypothesis certainly does not imply – as is so often misunderstood and misquoted – that '... [after] the first drink. . .relapse is automatic, inevitable and beyond control' (Littman, 1980). 'Lack of control' drinkers can often drink moderately for shorter or, more rarely, longer periods. In theory, therefore, there seems no reason why the great majority of alcoholics could not continue to drink in moderation perhaps indefinitely. In practice, however, under conditions and stresses of ordinary day-to-day living, so many unpredictable personal and social factors can act as internal and external cues activating the lack of control that relatively few such drinkers can realistically hope to achieve moderate drinking for longer than relatively short periods. Leaving aside the difficult-to-answer question why so many experienced clinicians only rarely if ever encounter a safe moderate drinker, we can base our conclusions on the estimates of 9–15% success made by protagonists of controlled drinking success as a basis (Pattison, 1976; Heather and Robertson, 1981). The price then paid by approximately nine out of ten alcoholics who attempt 'controlled drinking', in jeopardizing and undermining not only their own physical and mental health, but also (at least) the mental health of their spouse and children, hardly justifies the very risky, Russian roulette type of gamble. No-one would disagree with Pattison's (1966) statement that by itself 'abstinence is an inadequate criterion of health or of successful treatment in alcoholism', but at present, and until clear-cut answers can be given to the questions above, abstinence remains the most hopeful and reliable means of assisting both the drinker and his or her family towards achieving a healthy, satisfying, contented and useful life.

ACKNOWLEDGEMENTS

This chapter has been extended and revised from lectures presented at the 11th European Institute for the Prevention and Treatment of Alcoholism, Oslo, June 1965 (ICCA); the 30th International Congress on Alcoholism and Drug Dependence, Amsterdam 1972 (ICCA); the First International Medical Conference on Alcoholism, London, 1973 (Medical Council on Alcoholism); the 21st International Institute on the Prevention and Treatment of Alcoholism, Helsinki, June 1975 (ICCA); the Irish Branch of the Royal College of Psychiatrists' Meeting, Dublin, November 1979; and the First World Conference on Alcoholism, London, September 1981 (Charter Medical and ICCA).

The author and publishers are indebted to the organizers for their kind permission to use material presented at these conferences.

REFERENCES

Annaes, S. (1974). Alkoholisk kardiomyopati. *Ugesr. Laeg.*, **136**, 130

Anonymous (1981). What GPs can do for problem drinkers: a fresh approach. *Drug. Ther. Bull.*, **19**, 89

Armor, D. J., Polich, J. M. and Stambul, H. B. (1976). *Alcoholism and Treatment.* (Santa Monica: Rand Corporation)

Armor, D. J., Polich, J. M. and Stambul, H. B. (1978). *Alcoholism and Treatment.* (New York: John Wiley)

Arroyave, F. and McKeown, S. (1981). Controlled drinking – a perspective. *Br. J. Hosp. Med.*, **6**, 304

Bergman, H., Borg, S., Hindmarsh, T., Idestrom, C. M. and Mutzell, S. (1980). Computed tomography of the brain and neuropsychological assessment of male alcoholic patients. In Richter, D. (ed.) *Addiction and Brain Damage.* p. 201. (London: Croom Helm; Baltimore: University Park Press)

Chalmers, D. K. (1979). The alcoholic's controlled drinking time. *World Alcohol Project*, **2**, 18

Clare, A. W. (1977). How good is treatment? In Edwards, G. and Grant, M. (eds.) *Alcoholism – New Knowledge and New Responses.* p. 279. (London: Croom Helm)

Cohen, M., Liebson, I. A., Faillace, L. A. and Speers, W. (1975). Alcoholism: controlled drinking and incentives for abstinence. *Psychol. Rep.*, **28**, 575

Czypionska, A. and Demel, I. (1976). Kontrolliertes Trinken bei Alkohokranken. *Z. Klin. Psychol.*, **5**, 92

Davies, D. L. (1962). Normal drinking in recovered alcohol addicts. *Q. J. Stud. Alcohol*, **35**, 523
Davies, D. L. (1973). Implication for medical practice of an acceptable concept of alcoholism. In Kessel, N., Hawker, A. and Chalke, H. (eds.) *Alcohol – A Medical Profile. Proceedings of the First International Conference on Alcoholism.* p. 113. (London: B. Edsall)
Davies, D. L. (1979). Conversation with Davies, D. L. *Br. J. Addict.*, **74**, 239
Davis, M. (1980). Alcoholic liver disease: what the practising clinician needs to know. *Br. J. Addict.*, **75**, 19
Editorial (1975). *Lancet*, **1**, 152
Edwards, G. and Gross, M. M. (1976). Alcohol dependence; provisional description of a clinical syndrome. *Br. Med. J.*, **1**, 1058
Edwards, G. *et al.* (1977). *Alcohol-related disabilities.* (WHO Offset Publications, No. 32)
Emrick, C. D. (1974). A review of psychologically oriented treatment of alcoholism: I. The use of interrelationships of outcome criteria and drinking behaviour following treatment. *Q. J. Stud. Alcohol*, **33**, 523
Engle, K. B. and Williams, T. K. (1972). Effect of an ounce of vodka on alcoholics. *Q. J. Stud. Alcohol*, **33**, 1099
Ewing, J. A. (1973). Discussion. In Kessel, N., Hawker, A. and Chalke, H. (eds.) *Alcohol – A Medical Profile. Proceedings of the First International Medical Conference on Alcoholism.* p. 129. (London: B. Edsall)
Ewing, J. A. and Rouse, B. A. (1973). *Alcoholism (Zagreb)*, **9**, 64
Ewing, J. A. and Rouse, B. A. (1976). Failure of an experimental treatment programme to inculcate controlled drinking in alcoholism. *Br. J. Addict.*, **71**, 123
Gitlow, S. E. (1968). The pharmacological approach to alcoholism. In Bailey, M. B. (ed.) *Alcoholism and Family Casework, Theory and Practice.* p. 39. (New York: The Community Council of Greater New York)
Glatt, M. M. (1955). Treatment centre for alcoholics in a mental hospital. *Lancet*, **1**, 1318
Glatt, M. M. (1958). The English drink problem, its rise and decline through the ages. *Br. J. Addict.*, **54**, 51
Glatt, M. M. (1959). An alcoholic unit in a mental hospital. *Lancet*, **2**, 397
Glatt, M. M. (1961). Drinking habits of English (middle-class) alcoholics. *Acta Psychiatr. Scand.*, **37**, 88
Glatt, M. M. (1962). The abuse of barbiturates in the United Kingdom. *Bull. Narcot, (UN)*, **14**(2), 19
Glatt, M. M. (1965) The question of moderate drinking despite 'loss of control'. Paper presented at the Eleventh European Institute of Prevention and Treatment of Alcoholism, Oslo. Also *Br. J. Addict.* (1967), **62**, 267
Glatt, M. M. (1966). The 'loss of control' myth. *Lancet*, **1**, 1423
Glatt, M. M. (1970). *The Alcoholic and the Help He Needs.* (London: Priory)
Glatt, M. M. (1972). *Thirtieth International Congress on Alcoholism and Drug Dependence. Resumé*, Vol. 1. (Amsterdam)
Glatt, M. M. (1973). Loss of control. Extensive interdisciplinary borderland, not a sharp pharmacological borderline. In Kessel, N., Hawker, A. and Chalke, H. (eds.) *Alcoholism – A Medical Profile. Proceedings of The First International Medical Conference on Alcoholism.* p. 122. (London: B. Edsall)
Glatt, M. M. (1974). *A Guide to Addiction and its Treatment.* (Lancaster: MTP Press)
Glatt, M. M. (1975). Absolutism and alcoholism. *Lancet*, **1**, 447
Glatt, M. M. (1976). Alcoholism disease concept and loss of control revisited. *Br. J. Addict.*, **71**, 135

Glatt, M. M. (1979). Can alcoholics ever drink socially? *MIMS*, 15 March, 5
Glatt, M. M. (1980). The alcoholic and controlled drinking. *Br. J. Alc. Alcohol*, **15**(2), 48
Glatt, M. M. (1982). *Alcoholism*. (London: Teach Yourself Books)
Glatt, M. M. *et al.* (1978). Proceedings of a Conference, Jersey, December, 1977. *Age, Ageing*, **7** (Suppl.), 64
Goodwin, D. (1976). *Is Alcoholism Hereditary?* (New York: Oxford University Press)
Gottheil, E., Murphy, B. F., Skoloda, T. E. and Corbett, L. O. (1972). Fixed interval drinking decisions II. Drinking and discomfort in 25 alcoholics. *Q. J. Stud. Alcohol*, **33**, 325
Gross, M. M. (1973). Discussion. In Kessel, N., Hawker, A. and Chalke, H. (eds.) *Alcoholism – A Medical Profile. Proceedings of the First International Medical Conference on Alcoholism*. p. 129. (London: B. Edsall)
Heather, N. and Robertson, I. (1981). *Controlled Drinking*. pp. 29, 75, 105, 109, 200, 219, 231. (London, New York: Methuen)
Hodgson, R. J. (1980). The alcohol dependence syndrome: a step in the wrong direction. *Br. J. Addict.*, **75**, 255
Hodgson, R. J., Stockwell, T., Rankin, H. and Edwards, G. (1978). Alcohol dependence: the concept, its utility and measurement. *Br. J. Addict.*, **73**, 4
Hodgson, R. J., Rankin, H. J. and Stockwell, T. R. (1979). Alcohol dependence and the priming effect. *Behav. Res. Ther.*, **17**, 379
Hodgson, R. J. (1980). Treatment strategies for the early problem drinker. In Edwards, G. and Grant, M. (eds.) *Alcoholism Treatment in Transition*. p. 162. (London: Croom Helm)
Institute of Medicine (1980). *Alcoholism, Alcohol Abuse and Related Problems: Opportunities for Research*. p. 153. (Washington, DC: National Academy Press)
Jellinek, E. M. (1952a). The phases of alcohol addiction. *WHO Tech. Rep. Ser.*, **42**, 26
Jellinek, E. M. (1952b). Phases of alcohol addiction. *Q. J. Stud. Alcohol*, **13**, 673
Jellinek, E. M. (1960). *The Disease Concept of Alcoholism*. (New Brunswick: Hillhouse Press)
Keller, M. (1958). Alcoholism: nature and extent of the problem. *Ann. NY Acad. Sci.*, **133**, 820
Keller, M. (1972). On the loss of control phenomenon in alcoholism. *Br. J. Addict.*, **67**, 153
Keller, M. (1980). Psychological superstition and physical phallacy. *Br. J. Addict.*, **75**, 225
Kjolstadt, T. (1963). Further comment on Davies, D. L. 'Normal drinking in recovered alcohol addicts'. *Q. J. Stud. Alcohol*, **24**, 728
Leading article (1981). Minor brain damage and alcoholism. *Br. Med. J.*, **283**, 455
Lishman, W. A. (1981). Cerebral disorder in alcoholism syndromes of impairment. *Brain*, **104**, 1
Lishman, W. A., Ron, M. and Acker, W. (1980). Computed tomography of the brain and psychometric assessment of alcoholic patients – a British study. In Richter, D. (ed.). *Addiction and Brain Damage*. p. 215. (London: Croom Helm; Baltimore: University Park Press)
Littman, G. K. (1980). Relapse in alcoholism: traditional and current approaches. In Edwards, G. and Grant, M. (eds.). *Alcoholism Treatment in Transition*. p. 303. (London: Croom Helm)
Madden, J. S. (1979). *A Guide to Alcohol and Drug Dependence*. p. 114. (Bristol: John Wright)

Mann, M. (1968). *New Primer on Alcoholism.* 2nd Edn. (New York: Holt, Rinehart and Winston)
Martensen-Larsen, O. (1950). The significance of a low alcohol limen. *Br. J. Addict.*, **47**, 43
Marx, R. (1981). Fallstudie zum kontrollierten Trinken; zweifelhater Erfolgbei maximalem Aufwang. 27th International Institute of Prevention and Treatment of Alcoholism, Vienna, 15–19 June
Mello, N. K. and Mendelson, J. H. (1972). Drinking patterns during work-contingent and non-contingent alcohol acquisition. *Psychosom. Med.*, **34**, 139
Mendelson, J. H. (1964). Quoted in Paredes *et al.* (1977). 98
Merry, J. (1966). The 'loss of control' myth. *Lancet*, **1**, 1257
M. G. K. (1980). *Br. J. Alc. Alcohol*, **15**(1), 13
Murphree, H. N. (1976). Some possible origins of alcoholism. In Filstead, W. J., Rossi, J. J. and Keller, M. M. (eds.). *Alcohol and Alcohol Problems: New Thinking and New Directions.* p. 135. (Cambridge: Mass.: Ballinger)
Orford, J. and Edwards, G. (1977). *Alcoholism.* p. 105. (Oxford: Oxford University Press)
Paredes, A., Hood, W. R., Seymour, H. and Gollob, M. (1977). Loss of control in alcoholism: an investigation of the hypothesis, with experimental findings. In Pattison, E. M. *et al.* (ed.). *Emerging Concepts of Alcohol Dependence.* p. 96. (New York: Springer Verlag)
Pattison, E. M. (1966). A critique of alcoholism treatment concepts, with special reference to abstinence. *Q. J. Stud. Alcohol*, **27**, 49
Pattison, E. M. (1976). Nonabstinent drinking goals in treatment of alcoholism. A clinical typology. *Arch. Gen. Psychiatry*, **33**, 923
Pattison, E. M. and Headley, E. B. *et al.* (1977). In Pattison, E. M., Sobell, M. B. and Sobell, L. C. (eds.). *Emerging Concepts of Alcohol Dependence.* p. 120. (New York: Springer)
Pattison, E. M., Sobell, M. B. and Sobell, L. C. (1977). *Emerging Concepts of Alcohol Dependence.* p. 1. (New York: Springer)
Pittman, D. J. and Tate, R. J. A. (1969). A comparison of two treatment programmes for alcoholics. *Q. J. Stud. Alcohol*, **30**, 888
Portal, R. W. (1981). *Br. Med. J.*, **283**, 1202
Rosch, W. (1974). Die Wirkung von Alkohol und Nikotin auf den gastrointestinal Trakt. *Fortschr. Med.*, **92**, 316
Royal College of Psychiatrists (1979). *Alcohol and Alcoholism. Report of a Special Committee of the Royal College of Psychiatrists.* p. 130. (London: Tavistock)
Schukitt, M. A. *et al.* (1972). *Am. J. Psychiatry*, **128**, 1352
Smith, R. (1981). Treating alcohol problems: making ends meet. *Br. Med. J.*, **283**, 1043
Smithers, R. B. (1976). Personal letter accompanying booklet *Experimentation.* (New York: D. Smithers Foundation)
Wallace, J. (1979). Alcoholism and treatment revisited. *World Alcohol Project*, **2**, 3
Wessely, P., Hever, G. and Kryspin-Exner, K. (1973). Analyse der im Rahmen der Alkohol-krankheit auftretenden Anfalle aus dem Formenkreis der zerebral gesteuerten Anfalle. *Wien. Z. Nervenheilk.*, **31**, 63
WHO Expert Committee (1964). Expert committee on addiction producing drugs. *Thirteenth Report*, **273**, 9
WHO Expert Committee (1965). Drug dependence: its significance and characteristics. *Bull. WHO*, **32**, 721
Williamson, J. (1978). *Age, Ageing*, **7** Suppl., 68

7

Dependence and psychoactive drugs

John Marks

TERMINOLOGY

The term 'psychotropic substance', though widely used by the medical and lay public, and reasonably well understood by both groups, is one for which there is no fully accepted definition. Thus the United Nations Convention on Psychotropic Substances (1971) defines it as 'any substance, natural or synthetic, or any natural material in Schedule I, II, III or IV of the Convention'. Many would regard this as a rather restrictive definition.

It implies that a substance shall only be termed 'psychotropic' if it has a level of dependence liability, and social and public health problems which, compared with the level of therapeutic use, justify international control. This is clearly against the generally accepted much wider concept of the term, which was indeed accepted by the WHO Expert Committee on Drug Dependence (1970). They pointed out that many of the drugs covered within the broadly accepted use of the term 'psychotropic' do not produce dependence and that the restrictive use subsequently adopted by the United Nations could 'lead to confusion and misunderstanding'.

However since the Convention on Psychotropic Substances (1971) adopted the narrower sense of the term 'psychotropic' it is probably safer to use the term 'psychoactive' for the broader sense, namely: 'A substance with the capacity to produce ... central nervous system stimulation or depression, resulting in hallucinations or disturbances in motor function or thinking or behaviour or perception or mood....' (Convention on Psychotropic Substances, 1971).

Psychoactive, used in this sense, therefore, includes central nervous system depressant, stimulant and hallucinogenic drugs, whether or not they produce dependence. It would include alcohol and caffeine, and might be deemed to include nicotine. Although narcotics come within the broad definition they are dealt with elsewhere in the book and are therefore excluded.

THE CURRENT MEDICAL AND LAY REACTION TO THE USE OF PSYCHOACTIVE DRUGS

Over the past few years articles on psychoactive drugs have proliferated in both the medical and lay media. Many of these articles have been critical of the therapeutic value of this group of drugs and have concentrated on the problems. Terms like 'addiction', 'craving' and 'hooked' have been used. These are emotive terms with no clear relation to official definitions. While the risks are stressed, the benefits are almost ignored. All too often these articles are written by younger psychiatrists and journalists who have grown up only during the period of the availability of the modern psychoactive drugs. They have no memory of the life of the inpatient or outpatient mentally ill before such drugs became available. For those who can remember the period before the modern drugs, the benefits are still clear – despite current problems.

This is not to say that problems, particularly those related to dependence, do not occur with the majority of the psychoactive drugs. Few such drugs are entirely devoid of dependence liability. Some have a high abuse risk and no therapeutic value. The dependence liability of others is so large (for example, barbiturates, amphetamines) that they now have a negligible place in therapy. For others the liability is low and the risks must be balanced against the therapeutic benefits.

Another problem of psychoactive drugs is abuse within the 'street scene'. The psychoactive drugs that are abused to the greatest extent in the non-therapeutic situation are alcohol, tobacco and cannabis. These substances are considered in detail in other chapters of the book. By comparison the prescribable psychoactive drugs, whether stimulant or sedative, are much less widely abused and then usually as part of the mixed drug use that is the current pattern. This aspect of dependence of psychoactive drugs is considered later in this chapter.

THE MULTIFACTORIAL NATURE OF DEPENDENCE TO PSYCHOACTIVE DRUGS

The concept of a dependence-producing 'capacity' or 'potential' which resides in a drug itself has been questioned by some authorities in respect of drugs other than narcotics. These authorities suggest that it is more relevant to speak of 'dependence-prone individuals' who abuse a variety of substances and can develop dependence upon any or all of them. This has been described by Edwards (1967) in the case of alcohol. It can equally be applied to the group of drugs that the WHO Expert Committee on Dependence-producing Drugs (1964) classifies together with alcohol (barbiturates, non-barbiturate sedatives and tranquillizers).

It is apparent that within the field of psychostimulants and sedatives there is a contributory role exerted by the drug. Studies in both animals and man have demonstrated clear evidence of physical and psychological dependence when large doses are given for a prolonged period (Marks 1978; WHO Expert Committee on Drug Dependence, 1978; WHO Scientific Group, 1964, 1975). Moreover clinical reports on at least some of those who have become dependent during therapy reveal a previously normal personality. Various attempts have been made to express the liability risk of substances in quantitative form (WHO Expert Committee in Drug Dependence, 1978).

Nevertheless it is clear that there are several factors that lead to dependence on a drug in which the nature of the drug is only one of the elements, the others including the individual himself and his environment (WHO Scientific Group, 1975). The importance of environmental, personal and behavioural factors compared with pharmacological has been stressed by Fabre and Harris (1975). Berger (1972) even goes so far as to say 'there are no addictive drugs, only addictive people'. Although this, in my opinion, overstates the situation, it does stress the multifactorial nature of the problem.

ASSESSMENT OF DEPENDENCE LIABILITY OF PSYCHOACTIVE SUBSTANCES

Two World Health Organization Expert Committees (WHO Scientific Group, 1964, 1975) have reviewed the techniques for evaluating the dependence potential of drugs in general. The specific problem of the assessment of the dependence liability of psychotropic drugs was considered in the Twenty-first Report of the WHO Expert Committee on Drug Dependence (1978). Readers are advised to consult these publications for a detailed consideration of the techniques, their merits and problems. This present account only reviews the broad principles.

Both animal and human techniques are available; most of the former studies relate to physical dependence. Since the methods used in animal research determine factors that may or may not be related to factors for human dependence, they must of course be correlated with human experience to ensure that they have clinical validity. Ultimately, of course, the risk of dependence in patients using drugs under therapeutic conditions can only be determined during normal clinical usage. However, experience has shown that some of the experimental methods lead to valid assessment of the risk.

ANIMAL STUDIES

Despite the fact that the various substances demonstrate marked differences in their manifestations of dependence in man, animal tests for possible dependence follow a similar pattern for all substances.

PHARMACOLOGY AND TOXICOLOGY

A *sine qua non* of dependence production is that the substance shall have an effect on central nervous system activity. This can be demonstrated in single and multiple-dose pharmacological studies and such studies therefore form part of the testing procedure. Coupled with these pharmacological tests there can be biochemical investigations showing alteration of levels of transmitter substances (for example, the biogenic amines).

It is also valuable to examine the toxicological profile of the substance at this stage. Substances with unpleasant and immediate side-effects are less likely to be abused than those that do not show such properties.

During pharmacological studies various other phenomena commonly associated with dependence may become apparent. These include cross-tolerance with substances of known dependence liability, drug interactions, behaviour changes, particularly those of rapid onset, and rebound effects after stopping the drug.

STUDIES THAT SUGGEST PHYSICAL DEPENDENCE LIABILITY

Such studies can be divided into two classes: those in which the substance induces primary dependence in one or more animal species when administered on a chronic basis; and those in which the substance can be shown to substitute for one of known dependence liability in animals that have been made physically dependent on that agent. The present techniques have been reviewed recently (Thompson and Unna, 1977).

The primary induction of dependence with sedative and hypnotic drugs has been accomplished in various species, including rodents, cats and monkeys. It is important to establish the appropriate dose level and time interval to achieve the effect. During the administration it is possible with sedative compounds to demonstrate that the threshold to electrically and chemically induced convulsions is reduced. When the drug is stopped there is a lowering of the convulsion threshold and withdrawal signs are seen, the severity of which varies with the level of physical dependence. The signs of withdrawal from the sedative-hypnotics include convulsions, tremor and hyperirritability.

Substitution techniques for sedative-hypnotic drugs has usually been undertaken in animals previously made dependent on a barbiturate, and methods have been established for such trials in rodents, dogs and monkeys (WHO Expert Committee on Drug Dependence, 1978). It is important to realize that physical dependence has so far only been positively established for drugs that show central nervous system depressant activity. Hence the tests described above have no place in the study of stimulants or hallucinogens.

STUDIES THAT SUGGEST PSYCHOLOGICAL DEPENDENCE LIABILITY

It is currently held that psychoactive substances that demonstrate psychological dependence in man show reinforcement of drug-seeking and drug-taking behaviour in animals. Hence the majority of animal studies to predict psychological dependence liability involve self-administration techniques. These have now been established for a variety of species including rats, cats, dogs and monkeys (WHO Expert Committee on Drug Dependence, 1978). Most depend upon a lever-pressing stimulus for administration of the drug by intravenous or intragastric routes. Such reinforcing effects in animal studies have been demonstrated for both central nervous system depressants and stimulants, but the results are, to say the least, equivocal for hallucinogens.

As with the tests for physical dependence, so with the self-administration tests; the methods involve both primary progressive phenomena and cross-substitution. In some techniques the animals can choose between different drugs, so a preference rating for self-administration can be attempted. Of particular relevance to stimulant drugs are some of the drug discriminative procedures (Silverman and Ho, 1977).

RESULTS WITH THE DIFFERENT DRUG GROUPS IN ANIMAL STUDIES

Barbiturates and most sedatives show positive results in animal studies devised to demonstrate both physical and psychological dependence.

There are no convincing animal methods by which the dependence liability of *amphetamine*-type drugs can be assessed. The current methods involve behavioural studies demonstrating psychomotor stimulation and tolerance and reinforcement behaviour in self-administration studies.

Although *hallucinogens* are classified with the dependence-producing drugs for legislation purposes and are clearly drugs of abuse, there is little convincing evidence that they really have a dependence liability. It is therefore scarcely surprising that there are no clear predictive animal tests for these. Among the currently available drugs there is a measure of correlation between abnormal patterns of animal behaviour after drug administration and abuse potential in man, but there is no reason to believe that this would apply with new and further chemical classes of psychedelic drugs.

HUMAN STUDIES

The reports of adverse effects, by their very nature, must be anecdotal in the first instance, and this is also true of dependence. Although experimental production of dependence in volunteers was undertaken in the past, there are grave doubts about the ethics of such a procedure. This applies particularly to sedative–hypnotic compounds. In large doses these produce physical dependence in which withdrawal is characterized by convulsions and toxic psychosis. There is a significant level of morbidity, and indeed mortality, with withdrawal of such drugs. This therefore precludes such studies on an experimental basis. Moreover, very high doses are usually required to provoke dependence within a reasonable time-span and the validity of the observations for practical therapeutics is therefore in doubt. The ethical considerations covering attempted substitution, reinforcement techniques and preference rating of research compounds in known addicts are less clear, but such methods would in any case only give information relative to known and recognized types of dependence and not to a new class.

Current, natural medical and regulatory concern about dependence is likely to ensure that any compound with a dependence liability which manifests itself at the clinical trial stage does not reach the marketplace. This implies that in a practical therapeutic sense the dependence risk of new drugs is likely to be low and mainly determined by medical practitioners in isolated patients after long-term therapeutic use.

Specific facilities for reporting, investigating and recording reputed adverse reactions have now been established by most national authorities. Doctors should be encouraged to report any suspected dependence to these units. In addition the manufacturer should be informed; most research-based pharmaceutical companies have full facilities for correlating the available data and have a responsibility to determine the risk.

For any such assessment of the incidence of dependence under therapeutic conditions it is important to ensure that maximum information is recorded. The accuracy of the information should be independently cross-checked for each case as far as possible; those who are dependent are notoriously unreliable. Among information required is: the disorder that led to the administration of the drug; the age of the patient; previous use or abuse of drugs of potential dependence; current and previous levels of alcohol intake; the dose of the psychotropic prescribed; the dose of psychotropic actually taken; the length of administration.

It is, however, not sufficient to record the cases but to attempt to express the incidence relative to the extent of usage. This can be based upon prescription audits, patient audits, manufacturers' figures and official statistics (Marks, 1978). There is a measure of inaccuracy in each of these methods and they have different sources of error. There are, therefore, advantages in using several different measurements as cross checks.

PSYCHOTROPICS IN THE DRUG ABUSE SCENE

In the 'street drug scene' over the past decade a mixed pattern of abuse has been very common (Kryspin-Exner and Demel, 1975; Marks, 1982) and this is still true. The exact pattern depends on factors which include the main substance of dependence, the social class of the group (university students compared with 'skid row-ites') and national or local fads and fashions.

Some form of sedative compound is usually included in the mixture and the benzodiazepines are among the more commonly used sedatives.

Woody *et al.* (1975) found up to 40% of their narcotic addicts were 'diazepam users', although they stress that the proportion of this which is misuse or abuse is uncertain. This high figure is somewhat surprising, because when preference rating has been done the benzodiazepines are much lower than several other drugs (Du Pont, 1976). The high incidence may be representative only of the wide availability of the benzodiazepines as a result of their high safety factor. It is also very common to find that a psychostimulant is used within the mixture by such people.

It is often difficult to assess whether there is a true drug dependence for any individual drug in such patients due to the following factors:

(1) The primary dependence may relate to another drug, the sedative or stimulant being used in a secondary fashion to reduce the undesirable effects of the main drug (Marks, 1982). In this situation it is therefore acting in a beneficial fashion rather than as true drug abuse.
(2) It appears probable that the simultaneous ingestion of two drugs of potential dependence often increases the risk of each.
(3) The clinical manifestations of physical dependence to many of these drugs is similar, and it is difficult to be certain that the dependence relates to each of them. There are currently no practical methods for separating them with certainty.

When considering the abuse of any drug within the 'drug scene' one must be careful to distinguish the prime drugs of abuse that lead to medical and social deterioration, and those perhaps having some dependence liability, that are nevertheless mainly used for beneficial purposes. It appears that this latter type, which includes many of the newer tranquillizers, does not increase the danger to either the individual or the community.

One particular abuse which should perhaps be considered within the drug scene at present is solvent sniffing. The deliberate inhalation of volatile hydrocarbons used as solvents for glues, as paint thinners, nail polish removers, aerosol spray solvents, dry cleaning liquids and fire extinguishers is currently a not uncommon occurrence among children and adolescents. As with so many drug abuse problems there are marked differences in national patterns. High levels are currently reported from Japan, for example.

The sniffing of aerosol sprays is probably among the most dangerous practices for they may contain chemicals which can freeze the vocal cords and cause laryngeal spasm and asphyxiation. Glue solvent, the substance most commonly sniffed, is intrinsically less hazardous than most of the other substances. Sudden death from the inhalation of solvents is often due to cardiac arrhythmia precipitated by physical activity immediately after the inhalation. Later deaths can be due to the hepatotoxicity of some of the compounds. A related abuse seen in adults, particularly anaesthetists, is volatile anaesthetic sniffing, and petrol abuse is also prevalent.

THE JUVENILE DRUG ABUSER

There would appear to be two kinds of glue sniffers, as indeed there are two kinds of juvenile drug abusers in general. They comprise, on the one hand, the experimenters who try various drugs once or twice at the suggestion of their peers, perhaps as a demonstration of independence, but do not continue to indulge in the practice. On the other hand, there are the chronic users who use their drugs as an escape from boredom, their environment or parental neglect. By definition, the experimenters, though perhaps trying several different drugs of abuse on different occasions, do not *progress* from the so-called soft drugs (mainly psychotropics) to the hard drugs (mainly the narcotics). The experimenters form the larger group among juvenile drug abusers. How far progression is a major feature of juvenile chronic users is a matter of dispute.

Table 7.1 *List of substances in Schedule I of Convention on Psychotropic Substances (1971). The same Schedule applies in each case to the salts of the substances listed whenever the existence of such salts is possible*

INN	*Other non-proprietary or trivial names*	*Chemical name*
1.	DET	*N*, *N*-diethyltryptamine
2.	DMPH	3-(1,2-dimethylheptyl)-1-hydroxy-7,8,9,10-tetrahydro-6,6,9-trimethyl-6H-dibenzo [b,d] pyran
3.	DMT	*N*,*N*-dimethyltryptamine
4. (+)-Lysergide	LSD, LSD-25	(+)-*N*,*N*-diethyllysergamide (d-lysergic acid diethylamide)
5.	mescaline	3,4,5-trimethoxyphenethylamine
6.	parahexyl	3-hexyl-1-hydroxy-7,8,9,10-tetrahydro-6,6,9-trimethyl-6H-dibenzo [b,d] pyran
7.	psilocine, psilotsin	3-(2-dimethylaminoethyl)-4 hydroxyindole
8. Psilocybine		3-(2 dimethylaminoethyl)-indol-4-yl dihydrogen phosphate
9.	STP, DOM	2-amino-1-(2,5-dimethoxy-4-methyl) (phenylpropane)
10.	tetrahydrocannabinols, all isomers	1-hydroxy-3-pentyl-6a, 7, 10, 10a-tetrahydro-6,6,9-trimethyl-6-H-dibenzo [b,d] pyran
11. Piperidine	ICP	1-[1-(2-thienyl)cyclohexyl]piperidine
12. Pyrrolidine	PHP or PCPY	1-(1-phenylcyclohexyl) pyrrolidine
13.	PCE	*N*-ethyl-1-phenyl cyclohexylamine

HALLUCINOGENIC-TYPE DRUG DEPENDENCE

Substances of this type currently available are listed in Schedule I of the Psychotropic Substances Convention (Table 7.1). They include lysergide

(LSD), a semi-synthetic derivative of ergometrine; mescaline, an alkaloid derived from the peyotl cactus; psilocybin and psilocine from the mushroom *Psilocybe mexicana*; tryptamine derivatives DET and DMT; tetrahydrocannabinol, one of the active principles of cannabis and certain synthetic substances such as STP.

Over the centuries there has been extensive ritual use of hallucinogenic substances. The mistaken recreational use of some of these substances has been very common in recent years. The ingestion of many of these substances produce changes in mood, distortion in the perception of time, sights and sounds, depersonalization, auditory and visual hallucinations and a sense of unreality. In a proportion of those taking the hallucinogens a prolonged toxic psychosis indistinguishable from schizophrenia develops.

These substances have no therapeutic value and their use is dangerous. For this reason they are placed in the most highly controlled schedule of the Convention on Psychotropic Substances (1971). Although there is continuing abuse of these drugs by the susceptible user there is no true evidence of either psychological or physical dependence in the accepted sense. The most prevalent and important of the hallucinogenic drugs of abuse is cannabis, and this is considered in detail in Chapter 5.

THE DEVELOPMENT OF DEPENDENCE TO PSYCHOACTIVE DRUGS DURING THERAPY

It is clear that most, if not all, drugs that are active within the central nervous system can lead to dependence if given at high dosage for prolonged periods. This applies not only to drugs that are used within the abuse scene but also those that are used in therapy.

The therapeutic use of psychotropic substances is large and this use can be supported medically. Several recent studies have shown a level of significant psychiatric morbidity of some 20–30% in the population, of which about half is recognized by medical practitioners (Lader, 1980; Marks, 1980). Thus the level of use of psychotropics of about 10% accords with the recognized psychiatric morbidity level. This situation is not restricted to the 'industrially developed' countries, for in the developing world up to 10% of the general population, and a much higher proportion of those seeking medical help, are reported to be suffering from mental illnesses (Leading article, 1975). Approximately one-third of such patients (Marks, 1981) can only live a reasonable life within the community by continuing psychotropic drugs. This has nothing to do with dependence, more to reducing the level of incapacity due to the psychiatric disorder. It follows from this that approximately one adult in 25 to 30 is taking psychotropic drugs on a long-term basis with full medical justification. These therefore risk the development of dependence. This in no way justifies the continued administration of psychotropic drugs when they are no longer needed. Methods for reducing the risk of dependence development during treatment are considered on page 176.

THE PROBLEM OF THE DIAGNOSIS OF DEPENDENCE IN THERAPY

For the patient with a florid physical dependence that developed during treatment, and for the mixed drug user in the 'street scene' who visits one doctor after another in the hope of obtaining suppliers, there is no difficulty in reaching a diagnosis.

A significant proportion of patients, however, do not present a classical picture. For example, they may have been treated with a psychoactive drug for some months. There is probably no increase in the daily dose, but when discontinuation of treatment is suggested the patient resists the idea. Sudden withdrawal of the drug leads to nervousness, tremor, sweating, etc. These symptoms and signs are not only those of a mild withdrawal reaction in a dependent person, but are frequently those of which the patient originally complained and for which treatment was instituted. In consequence it is often difficult, and in some cases may be impossible, to distinguish a mild dependence from a return of a psychosomatic illness. Nor should the unwillingness of patients to give up therapy be regarded as absolute evidence of psychological dependence. A patient with angina pectoris who benefits from nitrates will frequently carry the pills long after the need for their use has gone – but this cannot be regarded as a psychological dependence in the *true* sense. Likewise, a patient with a severe anxiety state who knows that he or she experiences relief with a particular drug is equally keen to continue effective treatment.

A further complication is the 'rebound' phenomenon that occurs with psychoactive and other drugs (such as antihypertensives, adrenergic beta-blockers). When a psychoactive drug is involved dependence may be wrongly diagnosed. There are no absolute pathognomonic signs of mild dependence of the 'barbiturate type' but features which suggest mild dependence are: hypersensitive sensations; and fairly rapid onset of symptoms (within days – the return of psychosomatic symptoms is usually delayed for several days). Thus the diagnosis of dependence can only be made on the basis of the reaction after withdrawal of the drug. In the author's opinion, for therapeutic use of psychoactive substances five different types of reactions can be distinguished:

(1) The 'crutch' reaction – worry about the removal of a therapeutic substance which is known to be effective coupled with a continued supposed need for treatment. This reaction also occurs with drugs other than those with psychoactive properties.
(2) The 'rebound' reaction – the withdrawal of many drugs, including others than psychotropics (such as beta-adrenergic blocking agents) can lead to a temporary increase of the disorder.
(3) Return of the previous psychiatric disorder.
(4) True psychological dependence.
(5) True physical dependence.

DEPENDENCE LIABILITY OF PSYCHOTROPIC SUBSTANCES USED IN THERAPY

An overall assessment of the risk of psychological and physical dependence and abuse liability was made by Isbell and Chrusciel (1970). A summary of their assessment for the main drug groups used in therapeutics is shown in Table 7.2. Some of these drugs are now rarely used (for example, monoureides, sedative halogens, tertiary acetylenic alcohols, cyclic ethers). The high dependence and abuse liability of other drugs is now widely accepted (for instance, barbiturates, meprobamate and related compounds, methaqualone, amphetamines). Indeed for some of these the abuse liability is so high that their current use is very restricted (amphetamines, for example).

Table 7.2 *Listing of dependence liability of psychotropic substances used in therapeutics. (Based in part, and updated from Isbell and Chrusciel, 1970)*

	Abuse liability	*Medical and social problems*	*Extent of current world medical use*
Central nervous system depressants			
barbiturates	+ + +	+ + +	+ +
bromides	±	+	±
chloral hydrate	+ +	+	±
paraldehyde	±	+	±
meprobamate and derivatives	+ +	+	+
methaqualone	+ + +	+ +	+
benzodiazepines	+	+	+ + +
phenothiazines	0(?)	+	+ +
Central nervous system stimulants			
amphetamines	+ + +	+ + +	±
ephedrine and derivatives	0(?)	0(?)	+
piperidine appetite suppressants	+ +	+ +	+
Antidepressants			
MAOIs	0	+ +	±
tricyclics	0(?)	+	+ +

The dependence of some of the psychoactive drug groups that are currently used extensively is considered in detail below.

BARBITURATES

Barbiturates were used extensively in the past as hypnotics, as daytime sedatives and as anticonvulsants. It is now clear that the majority of the members of this chemical series have a high dependence and abuse liability, a risk increased by the high general level of tolerance that develops with barbiturates. However, the risks with barbiturates are wider than just those of dependence and abuse. Barbiturates are associated with many deaths due to overdosage, either alone or with alcohol, and they can lead to chronic intoxication.

NON-BARBITURATE HYPNOTICS

All such drugs studied to date show some dependence liability (see Table 7.2), and the effects of withdrawal are similar to those found with barbiturates. The risk associated with different substances shows wide variation; thus, for example, methaqualone has a very high abuse risk. However, the number of cases of dependence also varies with the therapeutic popularity of the drug and hence with the exposure level.

PHENOTHIAZINES

Phenothiazines have a very low dependence liability, indeed there is some doubt whether true dependence can develop with phenothiazines. Their therapeutic value lies in the psychoses, whereas other substances are used for the neuroses.

BENZODIAZEPINES

Since this group is so widely used and the dependence liability has been the subject of intense discussion, they are dealt with at greater length.

In an attempt to define the dependence liability of the benzodiazepines the author undertook a study of all the published cases of benzodiazepine dependence between 1960 and mid-1977 and attempted to quantify the liability. The details of the study have been published elsewhere (Marks, 1978) and the findings can therefore be summarized.

There were 118 publications on benzodiazepine dependence in which at least minimal information was included. Within these publications there were 458 cases where there was *a priori* evidence of dependence. Of these, 401 occurred in a clear drug abuse situation, and only 57 within a therapeutic situation. About 15 of these must be regarded as being very poorly documented; but of the 42 well-documented cases during therapy physical dependence was present in 24, and psychological dependence in 23.

To determine the various factors involved in the development of the dependence, the author examined in detail the reports which gave adequate information on dosage, duration of ingestion and concurrent taking of alcohol or other drugs. This amounted to 112 patients from the whole group of 458 (that is, those in both the abuse and therapeutic situations).

Based on this sample (Figure 7.1):

(1) 64 (about 60%) were taking other drugs or alcohol.
(2) 12 were receiving dosage under twice the accepted therapeutic level, 23 were taking a dosage between twice and four times the

normal level, and the remaining 78 were receiving more than four times the accepted therapeutic level.

(3) Only 14 cases received benzodiazepines for under 6 months, 20 between 6 months and a year, and 78 for over 1 year.

(4) In only 1 case in the 17 years' reports was a therapeutic dose, taken alone, for a period of less than 6 months, reported as causing dependence.

Any such figures of known dependence only have relevance in relation to the extent of usage. Hence the author estimated total benzodiazepine use, in terms of million patient-months, from prescription audits, patient audits, manufacturers' figures and official statistics. Coupling the number of reported cases with these figures of usage, it will be seen that the incidence of published reports is within the range of one case per 5–10 million patient-months at risk if one includes both the therapeutic and drug abuse situation. The risk during therapeutic use is probably less than one case per 50 million patient-months (Table 7.3).

Table 7.3 *Estimated incidence of benzodiazepine dependence from published reports. (Based on Marks, 1978)*

	United States	*Germany*	*United Kingdom*
Patient-month exposure (millions)	924	247	150
Published cases 1960–77	113	44	14
Unpublished, recorded cases 1960–77	–	54	14
Total recorded cases	–	98	28
Published cases incidence (million patient-months)	8.2	5.6	10.7
Recorded cases incidence (million patient-months)	–	2.5	5.3

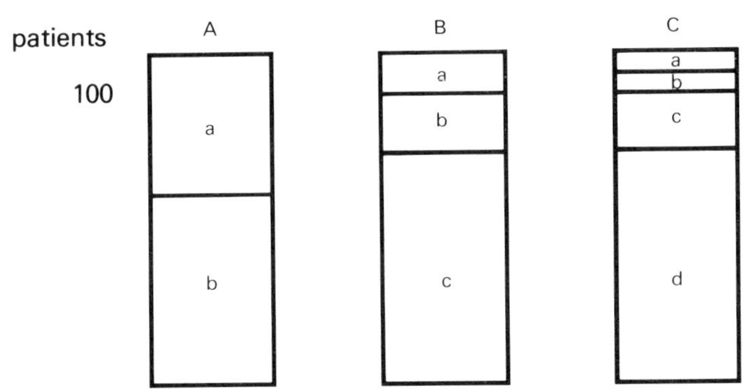

Figure 7.1 Factors that predispose to the development of dependence based on an analysis of 112 patients (from Marks, 1978). A (a) No other drugs used; (b) other drugs or alcohol also used. B (a) Less than twice therapeutic dose; (b) twice to four times therapeutic dose; (c) more than four times therapeutic dose. C (a) Less than 1 month administration; (b) between 1 and 6 months; (c) 6–12 months; (d) greater than 12 months

The information from published papers has been updated recently (Marks, 1982). This confirms the findings in the previous study (Marks, 1978), except that the proportion of publications that concern cases found to develop dependence while they were receiving accepted therapeutic doses of benzodiazepines has risen.

All benzodiazepines (whether 1,4 or 1,5 types) that have been commercially available for at least a year have been implicated. Differences between the incidence and time-course are considered below.

Hence it may be concluded that the risk for benzodiazepine dependence is very low in relation to their wide availability over a period of almost 20 years, and this accords with the conclusions of acknowledged world experts (Ayd, 1973; Glatt, 1974; Hollister, 1975; Kielholz, 1968; Kryspin-Exner and Demel, 1975). Published reports, however, do not necessarily represent the true incidence because the extent of reporting differs from one country to another and from one time-span to another. Ideally, a prospective study is needed in which a large number of patients with anxiety states or psychosomatic disorders, with no previous history of drug or alcohol abuse, are put on therapeutic doses of a benzodiazepine and then withdrawn at intervals of 3 months to determine the incidence and time-course of any development of dependence. Even were this medically feasible it would be ethically unsupportable.

The alternative study involves patients who have been on benzodiazepines for months or years and who are suddenly and deliberately withdrawn. Several such studies have been undertaken (Bowden and Fisher, 1981; Covi *et al.*, 1973; Kryspin-Exner and Demel, 1975; Laughren, 1981; Marks, 1981; Rickels, 1981; Rothstein, Cobble and Sampson, 1976; Tyrer, Rutherford and Huggett, 1981). The technical aspects of these studies are not always perfect: there is often no clear record of whether there is abuse of alcohol as well; the criteria for the selection of the cases is often not clear; ideally blood levels should be determined to make sure that therapy really has been withdrawn and that the patient is not taking either hoarded tablets or some received from other doctors.

Nevertheless, on the basis of the current studies some conclusions may be drawn about the incidence of withdrawal phenomenon when long-acting benzodiazepines are administered on a continuous basis (Table 7.4). Below 4–6 months the incidence of dependence is virtually nil unless there are additional factors involved (such as alcoholism) (Marks, 1981). At about a year the incidence of withdrawal phenomenon is probably about 3%, thereafter the incidence certainly rises and may reach high levels (Tyrer, Rutherford and Huggett, 1981).

The higher the unit dose the shorter is the exposure for reaching a risk-level, but the single most important factor appears to be the length of administration. Even at high doses for prolonged periods, a substantial proportion of users show no evidence of physical dependence. The factors involved are far from clear, but support the conclusion that there are dependence-prone individuals to benzodiazepines as well as to other substances (Edwards, 1967; WHO Expert Committee on

Dependence-producing Drugs, 1964). For benzodiazepines that are short-acting and rapid-acting, such as lorazepam, there is evidence that dependence can occur at a much earlier stage (under 3 months), that the overall level may be greater, and that reactions occur shortly after withdrawal and are more intense (Marks, 1982).

Table 7.4 *Current estimate of level of withdrawal phenomena with benzodiazepines*. Based on* continuous *treatment at therapeutic dosage with no additive factors (such as alcohol)*

	Long-acting	*Short and rapid-acting*
Less than 3 months	Nil	some
6 months	Rare	occasional
1 year	1–3% (perhaps up to 5%)	probably 5–10%
Over 1 year	increasing with duration (probably 10% +)	unknown – probably + +

**Note* This refers to withdrawal manifestations and does not equate with dependence

It is clear that with *continuous* prolonged ingestion, high levels of withdrawal symptoms can occur (Tyrer, Rutherford and Huggett, 1981). Whether all these represent dependence is open to doubt (see page 166). In Tyrer's study there was no positive control, so some of the manifestations may represent false reactions among patients led to expect difficulties with withdrawal by previous media reports.

However, there is a more important factor, namely that probably very few patients who are nominally taking continuous benzodiazepines are in fact actually taking them. Several researchers undertaking these studies have shown that it is very difficult to find patients who have maintained a steady dosage for several months. The majority seem to use these drugs, either by direction or in practice, in an 'on demand' manner, adjusting the dose up or down according to their current degree of distress. In one such study (Bowden and Fisher, 1981), although those selected were nominally taking continuous doses, the actual administration of standard doses resulted in higher blood levels and lower anxiety levels.

STIMULANTS

Dependence and abuse liability with dexamphetamine is very high and it is now rarely used in therapy. Other stimulants also show substantial risk of abuse, though for many it is perhaps less than that with dexamphetamine. Their therapeutic use is accordingly restricted.

TRICYCLIC ANTIDEPRESSANTS

Tricyclic antidepressants are not normally associated with dependence risk. However, recent reports (Gawin and Markoff, 1981; Mirin, Schatzberg and Creasey, 1981; Stern and Mendels, 1980) have appeared of reactions after the withdrawal of various tricyclic antidepressants, some taking the form of panic anxiety, others of hypomania. It appears that this is more likely to represent a rebound effect than true dependence.

SOCIAL IMPLICATIONS OF DEPENDENCE ON PSYCHOTROPIC DRUGS

The presence of social problems among those who are either excessive users or abusers of psychotropic drugs does not necessarily imply that the problems are caused by the consumption of the drug. The use of the drug, whether this be legally or illegally procured, may itself be a response to social difficulties already encountered by the individual. It is therefore important to appreciate the nature of this relationship and take account of it when social problems are being considered.

Illicit abuse of many psychoactive drugs may give rise to social difficulties within the narrow sphere of the group that directly surrounds the individual, and in the wider sphere of the community at large. Changes in interpersonal relationships that stem from use of some such drugs is an incontrovertible fact, but whether they are regarded as social problems depends on the views of the community, both small and large. This in its turn varies from one religion or ethos to another and, in the same community, from one generation to another. Consider, for example, the reaction of the community to the gin-sodden biddies of Hogarth cartoons, the laudanum-takers of the Victorian era, the hashish of the Middle East, opium of China and psilocybin of the Central Americas. These substances have often been of considerable economic or social importance to the societies in which their use has been permitted or even encouraged. It is, in fact, often difficult to distinguish between accepted cultural use and abuse of the same drug in a community, because as social patterns of behaviour change use can be regarded as abuse.

Although it may be difficult to distinguish all the social effects of psychotropic drug abuse, some problems that they cause can be recognized. These include economic losses for the subject and his circle, deteriorating family and social relationships, sometimes criminal behaviour in order to acquire the drug, and increased use of social and medical services. Nevertheless, the social costs of psychotropic drug abuse are widely regarded as being far less than those of the narcotics. To these social costs must also be added the public health costs of problems such as road traffic and industrial accidents, overdose deaths or morbidity, and toxic psychoses and other mental and physical disorders.

The social and public health cost is not uniform from one drug to another, for it is greatly influenced by the exact nature of the problems associated with the individual drug. Thus the barbiturates, for example, with their pronounced sedative effects and high suicide potential, carry a substantial social and public health cost. It is clear that all psychotropic drugs have some social costs. The International Convention for Psychotropic Substances (1971), which controls psychoactive substances, bases its consideration of the need for and type of control *inter alia* on the balance between the social costs and the therapeutic value of the substance.

Although all psychotropics have some social cost it should not be supposed that the abuse of psychotropic drugs can be totally avoided. Throughout the whole of recorded history there has probably never been an age in which people did not make use of some form of psychotropic substance. Although everyone is agreed that the best answer would be a society in which none of the members resorted to the use of such agents, this must be regarded as a utopian dream.

We must expect that in our non-utopian society the majority of the community will abuse some substance, whether this be a drug, alcohol or tobacco. In addition, there will always be socially inadequate personalities whose abuse of psychotropic drugs will be well above the norm. Hence some measure of social cost is inherent in the existence of any psychoactive substance. But the neuroses have their own social and public health costs, and for some the social cost may be large (for example, reduced work capacity and suicide in depression). Thus there can be social and public health benefits from the appropriate medical use of psychoactive medicines.

Many hundreds of studies have demonstrated the value for psychoactive substances in the relief of a wide range of psychiatric disorders, and there can be little doubt of their therapeutic value when they are used appropriately. Probably the main problem with the medical use of psychoactive drugs lies in their use when a wrong diagnosis has been made. Those who have seen the social problems associated with psychiatric illnesses and the improvement that results from correct treatment, can have little doubt that the rational use of psychotropic substances has clear social benefit. But the existence of this social benefit is not universally accepted. Even today it is only in the most sophisticated communities that mental illness is looked upon, like physical illness, as a disease and not as a cause for shame.

The very availability of psychotropic drugs has produced an ambivalent approach by society. On the one hand, there is the greater tolerance towards mental illness and its acceptance, but on the other hand a great hostility towards behavioural disorders caused by those drugs when their manifestations are contradictory to the accepted cultural model. Thus society tolerates certain drugs (tobacco, for instance) that on the basis of objective evidence can be shown to produce physical ills of great medical and social danger, but is hostile to others where evidence of iatrogenic social problems is largely based upon subjective emotions.

Thus there are socially acceptable diseases and socially acceptable drugs with no clear and rational basis for the division. In our current social pattern the neuroses and psychotropic drugs are still largely socially unacceptable, and tolerated as a necessary evil rather than lauded as a great medical and social benefit. Society's approach to mental illness is still broadly 'shake yourself out of it'.

There is an idea that the use of psychotropic drugs is 'bad and contributes to moral decline'. That to take them represents 'a weakness, a lack of self-control and self-reliance', and to prescribe them is to foster a sick society. Klerman (1972) has spoken of 'pharmacological Calvinism' and Blackwell (1973) of the 'puritan ethic' that 'patients should tolerate depression or anxiety and that medication for this end is to misuse it'. Both these writers have condemned this view as have many others including Abrahamson (1976) and Hollister (1975). Perhaps one of the best expressions of the contrary view is that by Morrison (1974). 'Rational, responsible use of psychotropic drugs to relieve even ill-defined psychological disorders should not be considered as a craven surrender to human weakness. There is nothing really noble about needless suffering.'

A greater medical and social dilemma exists over the chronic administration of psychotropic drugs. It is quite clear that their major use should be on a short-term basis to relieve the acute phase of mental illness, that like all medication they should be withdrawn as soon as possible, and that their long-term continuous administration leads to dependence in a significant proportion of those treated. Nevertheless it is apparent that a group of mentally ill patients exist who cannot achieve a socially acceptable existence unless they are receiving psychotropic medication. In the author's opinion the doctor has the moral and medical duty to discuss the pros and cons of continued therapy fairly with such patients, but to provide treatment if this is requested by the patient after he or she has been given the relevant information. Notwithstanding this, the patient and doctor should thoroughly review the situation at regular intervals or move to intermittent treatment to cover the worst periods of the illness.

REDUCTION OF DEPENDENCE TO THE PSYCHOTROPICS

Efforts to reduce psychotropic drug dependence can be considered under three headings: legislation to reduce illicit supplies and handling; reducing demand in the illicit-use field; and reducing demand in therapeutic use.

LEGISLATION TO REDUCE ILLICIT SUPPLIES AND HANDLING

At the national and international level there are restrictions on the supply and movement of drugs recognized as having a dependence liability. For those drugs where there is an international abuse situation and no therapeutic value (such as the hallucinogens) international control is tight and the substances are included in Schedule I of the United Nations Convention on Psychotropic Substances (1971) (see Table 7.1). At the other end of the scale are the psychoactive substances where there is extensive and justified therapeutic use, limited risk of dependence and no international illicit traffic. Such medicines are normally covered by national prescription legislation.

Table 7.5 *Summary of the main provisions of the four Schedules of the Convention on Psychotropic Substances (1971)*

	Schedule I	*Schedule II*	*Schedule III*	*Schedule IV*
Medical and scientific use	strict controls on very limited use	prescription	prescription	prescription
Manufacture and trade	special licence and very strict supervision	licence and control	licence and control	licence and control
Export and import	very strict controls on all movements	tight controls	recording and controls	recording and controls
Record-keeping and information to control bodies	careful records of all transactions available to authorities	careful records of all transactions available to authorities	summary records kept and supplied to authorities	trade records kept and supplied to authorities

Between these extremes are substances with a varying level of therapeutic value, risk of dependence, social problems and international illicit traffic, and these are covered by Schedules II, III and IV of the International Convention on Psychotropic Substances (1971). The full significance of the terms of this Convention are beyond the scope of this book but an outline of the main provisions are shown in Table 7.5. The inclusion or exclusion of substances from the Schedules or any change of Schedule is decided by the United Nations Commission on Narcotic Drugs, based upon the medical and scientific advice of the World Health Organization through its Expert Committee on Drug Dependence.

Treatment, rehabilitation or social reintegration of those who are dependent are in theory recognized among the most important elements in drug abuse control by reducing demand and are so stated in the Convention (Article 20). Nevertheless, in practice, due to lack of adequate funds and adequate methods of treatment, the emphasis tends to be placed more on methods of reducing *supply* than on reducing *demand*.

Examination of the official statistics of the level of illicit movement and use of narcotics makes it clear that this type of legislation is not, in itself, an adequate means of containing the problem. The balance of benefit that results from such international controls, based upon control of movement and supply, remains a matter for discussion. Protagonists of the controls point at the high level of seizures effected by the authorities and the consequent loss of the supplies to the users; antagonists suggest that the imposition of controls can itself lead to a subculture of users bound together by a resistance to authority, and to the stimulation of increased demand by shortage and the development of an illegal community to supply that demand at inflated prices and profits.

It is clear that those drugs that produce social and public health ills and are the subject of illicit international trading should be dealt with by strict international controls. However, if controls are spread too broadly it becomes impossible to enforce them and the whole basis of the law is weakened.

REDUCING DEMAND IN THE ILLICIT USE FIELD

As we have noted above, the reduction of demand by the treatment, rehabilitation and social reintegration of those dependent on drugs is accepted as an important method for reducing demand for such drugs. The real problem lies not in acceptance of the concept but in the absence of really effective techniques for effecting long-lasting abstinence, and in the costs involved. Numerous techniques have been and are being tried; indeed the number and variety of the current methods are a clear indication that there is no really successful method. The success rate is probably, at best, under 50%.

REDUCING DEMAND IN THERAPEUTIC USE

Since therapeutic use implies prescription by doctors, it follows that reduced demand in this area can be achieved by teaching doctors how best to use psychotropic drugs. This must be an ongoing educational process at both undergraduate and postgraduate levels as the range of drugs, their merits and difficulties changes rapidly. The main general principles that should reduce the level of dependence are:

(1) By the better selection of patients for psychotropic therapy. It is important to remember that not all patients with neurotic illnesses need drug treatment. Many such illnesses are self-limiting and of short duration and drugs are not always necessary (Rickels, 1981). It is also important to remember that patients who have been or are dependent on other drugs or alcohol show a greater tendency to dependence on psychotropic drugs, which should therefore be used with even greater caution (Marks, 1978).

(2) By careful selection of the drug to be used in the individual case. It is important to stress that some at least of the long-term, high-dosage, therapeutically ineffective but potentially dependence-provoking prescription of anxiolytics stems from the failure to recognize the concomitant existence of depression.

(3) By recognition that drugs form only one part, albeit a valuable part, of the total patient care. Psychoactive agents should be prescribed only after listening to the patient, assessing whether the cause can be removed, what effect the disorder will have on behaviour, and how best the various therapeutic procedures can be combined.

(4) By withdrawal of drug therapy as soon as this is therapeutically feasible.

CONCLUSIONS

Few if any psychotropic drugs are totally devoid of liability to produce psychological and/or physical dependence. All such drugs are liable to overuse and abuse. The level of dependence risk and the social costs inherent in the overuse differ from one drug to another.

Decisions about the use of these drugs should involve a consideration of the balance between the risk and social cost of dependence against the therapeutic merits of the drug and the medical needs of the patient. In all such decisions it is important to realize that drugs are only one part of the treatment of mental illness and should always be used with care and discontinued as soon as possible.

The control of psychotropic drugs is now exercised under the Convention on Psychotropic Substances (1971), with four Schedules based on the therapeutic value and liability risk.

REFERENCES

Abrahamson, A. (1976). Psychotropic drug use: fallacies and a paradox. *Psychol. Med.*, **6**, 529

Ayd, F. (1973). Patterns, range and effects of misused psychotropic substances in North America today. *Med. J. Aust.*, **60**, Suppl. 4, 27

Berger, H. (1972). There are no addictive drugs, only addictive people. *Postgrad. Med.*, **51**, 269

Blackwell, B. (1923). Psychotropic drugs in use today: the role of diazepam in medical practice. *J. Am. Med. Assoc.*, **225**, 1637

Bowden, C. L. and Fisher, J. G. (1981). Diazepam. The question of long-term therapy and withdrawal reactions. *Drug Ther. Suppl.*

Convention on Psychotropic Substances (1971). (New York: United Nations)

Covi, L., Lipman, R. S., Pattison, J. H., Derogates, L. R. and Uhlenhruth, E. H. (1973). Length of treatment with anxiolytic sedatives and response to their sudden withdrawal. *Acta Psychiatr. Scand.*, **49**, 51

Du Pont, R. L. (1976). Polydrug abuse and the maturing national drug abuse data base. *Ann. NY Acad. Sci.*, **281**, 311

Edwards, G. (1967). Personality and addiction. *Harvard J. Penal Ref.* **12**, 136

Fabre, L. F. and Harris, R. T. (1975). Clinical considerations in the abuse of anti-anxiety and antidepressant drugs. In F. Kapan *et al.* (eds.) *Hypnotics, Methods of Development and Evaluation.* p. 283 (New York: Spectrum)

Gawin, F. H. and Markhoff, R. A. (1981). Panic anxiety after abrupt discontinuation of amitriptyline. *Am. J. Psychiatry*, **138**

Glatt, M. M. (1974). *A Guide to Addiction and its Treatment.* Lancaster: MTP Press

Hollister, L. E. (1975). Drugs for emotional disorders. Current problems. *J. Am. Med. Assoc.*, **234**, 942

Isbell, H. and Chrusciel, T. L. (1970). Dependence liability of 'non-narcotic' drugs. *Bull. WHO*, **43**, Suppl.

Kielholz, P. (1968). Gesamtschwerzersche Enquete Ueber die Haeufigkeit das Medikamenten-Missbrauches. *Schweiz. Arzneitz*, **49**, 1077

Klerman, G. L. (1972). Psychotropic hedonism versus pharmacological Calvinism. *Hastings Center Rep.*, **2**, 1

Kryspin-Exner, K. and Demel, I. (1975). The use of tranquilizers in the treatment of mixed drug abuse. *Int. J. Clin. Pharmacol. Biopharm.*, **12**, 13

Lader, M. (1980). The present status of benzodiazepines in psychiatry and medicine. *Arzneim. Forsch.*, **30**, 910
Laughren, T. P. (1981). Diazepam. The question of long-term therapy and withdrawal reactions. *Drug Ther. Suppl.*
Leading article (1975). Mental health in developing countries. *Br. Med. J.*, **4**, 187
Marks, J. (1978). *The Benzodiazepines – Use, Overuse, Misuse, Abuse.* Lancaster: MTP Press
Marks, J. (1980). The benzodiazepines – use and abuse. *Arzneim. Forsch.*, **30**, 898
Marks, J. (1981). Diazepam. The question of long-term therapy and withdrawal reactions. *Drug Ther. Suppl.*
Marks, J. (1982). Benzodiazepines – use, misuse and abuse. *Thai Med. J.* (In press)
Marks, J. (1982). *The Benzodiazepines – for Good or Evil.* (In press)
Mirin, S. M., Schatzberg, A. F. and Creasey, D. E. (1981). Hypomania and mania after withdrawal of tricyclic antidepressants. *Am. J. Psychiatry*, **138**, 87
Morrison, A. B. (1974). Government control over psychotropic drugs. In R. Cooperstock (ed.). *Social Aspects and Medical Use of Psychotropic Drugs.* Toronto: Addiction Research Foundation
Rickels, K. (1981). Diazepam. The question of long-term therapy and withdrawal reactions. *Drug Ther. Suppl.*
Rothstein, E., Cobble, J. C. and Sampson, N. (1976). Chlordiazepoxide. Long-term use in alcoholism. *Ann. NY Acad. Sci.*, **273**, 381
Silverman, P. B. and Ho, B. T. (1977). Characterization of discriminative response control by psychomotor stimulants. In H. Lal (ed.). *Discriminative Stimulus Properties of Drugs*, p. 107. New York: Plenum Press
Stern, S. L. and Mendels, J. (1980). Withdrawal symptoms during the course of imipramine therapy. *J. Clin. Psychiatry*, **41**, 66
Thompson, T. and Unna, K. R. (eds.) (1977). *Predicting the Abuse Dependence of Stimulant and Depressant Drugs.* Baltimore: University Park Press
Tyrer, P., Rutherford, D., Huggett, T. (1981). Benzodiazepine withdrawal symptoms and propranolol. *Lancet*, **1**, 520
WHO Expert Committee on Dependence-Producing Drugs (1964). *Thirteenth Report, Annex 1. WHO Tech. Rep. Ser.* **No. 273**, Geneva
WHO Expert Committee on Drug Dependence (1970). *Seventeenth Report. WHO Tech. Rep. Ser.* **No. 437**, Geneva
WHO Scientific Group (1964). *Evaluation of Dependence-producing Drugs. Report WHO Tech. Rep. Ser.* **No. 287**, Geneva
WHO Scientific Group (1975). *Evaluation of Dependence Liability and Dependence Potential of Drugs. Report WHO Tech. Rep. Ser.* **No. 577**, Geneva
WHO Expert Committee on Drug Dependence (1978). *Twenty-first Report. WHO Tech. Rep. Ser.* **No. 618**, Geneva
Woody, G. E., Mintz, J., O'Hare, K., O'Brien, C. P., Greenstein, R. A. and Hargrave, E. (1975). In *Problems in Drug Dependence, 37th Ann. Meet. Washington, May 1975*, p. 1144. Washington, DC: National Academy of Science

8

The nature and treatment of cigarette dependence

Martin Raw

INTRODUCTION

Although prevalence of smoking in Britain is falling (Capell, 1978) smokers still make up 46% of the adult population (Office of Population Censuses and Surveys, 1978). This represents about 18 million smokers, and about 95 000 of these are estimated to die prematurely each year as a result of smoking (Wald, 1978). Smoking thus remains a very serious health problem in Britain, a continuing drain on the resources of both the health services and industry, and yet progress in reducing smoking-related disease, and smoking itself, is slow. There are many reasons for this: lack of real commitment from the government, the pleasure some smokers get from smoking, and the fact that many of them find it difficult to stop. Undoubtedly the 'addictiveness' of tobacco smoking is an important factor, although this should not be thought of in the narrow sense of so-called physical dependence. Tobacco dependence is a social, economic, psychological and physiological phenomenon.

THE NATURE OF CIGARETTE DEPENDENCE

Cigarette smoking is clearly a very strong 'addiction' or dependence. McKennell and Thomas (1967) showed that only 2% of smokers were able to limit themselves to occasional smoking, and that less than 15% were able to stop smoking permanently before the age of 60. They also found that 75% of smokers had either tried to stop smoking or said they wanted to stop. While 'I want to stop smoking' might include a wide range of motivation to stop, from 'I would like to stop if it were easy to do so' to 'I am desperate to stop and would do anything to succeed', 75%

represents about 13 million smokers, of whom several million at least must genuinely wish to stop. While this study is now somewhat out of date, strong evidence remains that many smokers still want to stop smoking, and feel they cannot do so without help. When in October 1977 a television programme broadcast to an estimated five million viewers offered smokers a free antismoking kit, designed to stop them smoking, nearly 500 000 people rang or wrote asking for the kit (Raw and van der Pligt, 1981). The low success rates at smoking-withdrawal clinics (Raw, 1978) also testifies to the dependence potential of cigarette smoking, and at an addiction clinic in London, drug users rated tobacco as their most needed drug, over heroin, methadone, amphetamine, barbiturate, LSD, cannabis, alcohol, tea and coffee (Blumberg, 1974).

In models of smoking the mechanisms accounting for onset are conventionally distinguished from those accounting for maintenance. The evidence above shows that cigarette smoking is a powerful dependence, but children do not take up smoking because of this, or even for its physiological effects, which are usually unpleasant at first. The onset of smoking, most commonly in adolescence, is explained by psychological and social factors. They try cigarettes through curiosity, the assertion of independence, or rebelliousness and are influenced by their parents' or friends' smoking. The number of friends smoking is one of the most powerful single factors (Bewley, Day and Ide, 1973; Bynner, 1969). These factors are strong enough to overcome the initial unpleasant side-effects of smoking and establish it as a regular behaviour. The MRC-funded study of smoking in Derbyshire schoolchildren (Bewley *et al.*, 1980), showed that by the age of 10–11, 7% of boys and 2½% of girls were regular smokers (one cigarette a week or more).

Once established, smoking is maintained by a variety of factors. These include the positive (or useful to the smoker) effects of nicotine (Stepney, 1980), the unpleasant effects of cigarette withdrawal (Raw, 1978) and, by implication, of withdrawal from nicotine, the social use of smoking (Stepney, 1980) and its relative cheapness (compared with 1950 prices) (Russell, 1973) and widespread availability. There is much evidence on the role of nicotine. Nicotine has a powerful effect on many body functions, including increasing heart rate, blood pressure and stroke volume, increasing cortical arousal and decreasing peripheral blood flow. It can also cause relaxation of some muscles and affect absorption of food from the gut. There is evidence that heavy smokers smoke in such a way as to regulate the nicotine level in their blood (Russell, 1980). There is little correlation between the nicotine yields of cigarettes, and blood nicotine concentrations in smokers (Russell *et al.*, 1980), which suggests that in regular smokers the pattern of smoking is determined not by the cigarette, but by the need to maintain an optimal blood nicotine concentration. There is also evidence, reviewed by Russell (1976), that when smokers are getting nicotine from another source (from chewing nicotine gum, or intravenously) they smoke fewer cigarettes.

These facts strongly suggest that nicotine is an important factor in explaining how and why smokers smoke, and it is significant that tobacco has never been used except in a way which allows absorption of nicotine into the bloodstream. However, not enough research has been done yet to determine the relative importance of pharmacological and psychosocial factors in light smokers. It seems likely that heavier smokers are more nicotine-dependent, and that lighter smokers smoke more for psychological and social reasons. The problem, however, with any such typologies of smoking (or motives for smoking), or of smokers, is that they seek to categorize, and in doing so to oversimplify. This is not easily done with smoking. Firstly, because both pharmacological and psychological motives for smoking are found in most smokers; few smokers are either purely dependent on nicotine, or purely social smokers. Secondly, because by concentrating on a concept like nicotine dependence, we are encouraged to think of tobacco dependence as an established, mainly physical condition, which, by implication, has a treatment or cure. But there is no 'cure' for cigarette 'addiction', and those dependent on cigarettes have to work very hard to change their behaviour. To call smoking an 'addiction' explains little. What is 'addiction'?

Smoking is a complex behaviour, and the actions of nicotine are varied. There is evidence that smokers use smoking to manipulate their level of arousal, in other words, that smoking is used by smokers as a (psychological) tool. There is also evidence that smoking is used to control stress and tension and that it is especially important in this respect socially (Stepney, 1980). These motives for smoking are not alternatives to dependence. Dependence could be said to encompass them all, as well as avoidance of physical and psychological withdrawal symptoms. To be dependent on something implies difficulty in doing without it. Cigarette smokers find it difficult to do without smoking for all these reasons: because it can be psychologically rewarding, physiologically rewarding, socially useful, painful to give up, and because cigarettes are so easy to obtain. Only recognition of this complexity will lead to a realistic approach to cigarette withdrawal, called in this chapter the treatment of cigarette dependence for descriptive convenience, not for theoretical reasons.

Stopping smoking involves changing many deeply ingrained patterns of behaviour and takes a long time. Individuals can be helped by specific 'treatments' like nicotine replacement, but must also invest time and effort of their own. Social change, as well as changes in the cost and distribution of tobacco are important adjuncts to this.

THE TREATMENT OF CIGARETTE DEPENDENCE

Tobacco smoking has never been an entirely acceptable custom in Britain. In 1857 the correspondence columns of the *Lancet* testified to grave concern, on the part of doctors, about the symptoms of nicotine poisoning in cigar-smoking patients. Attempts to help people stop smoking predate the first publications on smoking and lung cancer, and predate by many years more widespread acceptance of the dangers of smoking. A study on the 'control of the tobacco habit' was published by Dorsey in 1936, 10 years before a study by the psychoanalyst, Edmund Bergler (1946). The first smoking withdrawal clinic in Britain was opened in Salford in 1958, 4 years before the first report of the Royal College of Physicians, entitled *Smoking and Health*, after which smoking clinics became commoner. However in 1980 there were still only about 50 clinics in the whole of England and Wales, a figure which perhaps reflects official reluctance to recognize the strength of cigarette dependence.

SMOKING WITHDRAWAL CLINICS

Smoking withdrawal clinics have offered help to unselected (self-selected) smokers who walk in asking for help. Most have emphasized a group therapy approach. Apart from drug therapy specific treatments take second place to the dissemination of health information, group discussion and mutual support, and general advice on how to resist the urge to smoke. These clinics have achieved fairly consistent results and establish a baseline success rate for smoking withdrawal treatment. They have achieved a success rate (total abstinence) at 1-year follow-up of roughly 15–20%. Although they achieve a much higher short-term success rate, with up to 80% stopping smoking during treatment, most clients relapse during the first few months after treatment. Numerous studies show this pattern of outcome (Ejrup, 1964; McFarland *et al.*, 1964; Ross, 1967. Schwartz and Dubitzky, 1968) and they illustrate an important point: it is easy for smokers to stop smoking, but difficult for them to remain abstinent. It is important to bear this in mind when claims are made for high success rates using new stop-smoking methods. Commercial hypnotists, for instance, sometimes claim a success rate of 80–90%, which actually refers to the proportion of people claiming abstinence *straight after treatment*, not at 1 year follow-up.

DRUG THERAPY

Knowledge that tobacco contains nicotine led to drug therapy being tried very early in the search for an effective withdrawal aid. Two kinds of drug therapy have been investigated. Firstly tranquillizers have been used to relieve withdrawal symptoms (especially tension) but with little success (Bartlett and Whitehead, 1957; Turle, 1958; Whitehead and Davies, 1964). There is even some evidence than tranquillizers are worse than placebos, and actually hinder tobacco withdrawal (Schwartz and Dubitzky, 1968). The second approach to drug therapy has involved the use of nicotine substitutes, usually lobeline (*Lobelia inflata*), which shares many physiological properties with nicotine (Davison and Rosen, 1972). Again, there is no evidence that lobeline aids tobacco withdrawal over and above its placebo effect (Davison and Rosen, 1972; Dorsey,

1936; Edwards, 1964; Ford and Ederer, 1965; Merry and Preston, 1963). Undoubtedly one of the main reasons for the ineffectiveness of lobeline is that it does not mimic the effects of nicotine closely enough.

Nicotine itself has been used as a substitute for tobacco smoking, and the results of this work are reviewed under a separate section, page 187.

HYPNOSIS

'Although there are many clinical reports available there is almost no good research evidence attesting to the effectiveness of hypnosis in the elimination of smoking behaviour' (Johnson and Donoghue, 1971). This conclusion remains valid for two principal reasons. The first is the poor design of most clinical trials using hypnosis and the second is the difficulty of defining hypnosis. What is hypnosis? Is a trance necessary? Such a wide variety of procedures is reported in the literature that the only thing some have in common is the use of the word 'hypnosis' to describe them. It may be, of course, that hypnosis achieves its effect through support and the placebo effect of the word itself, and careful reading of the literature suggests a definition of hypnosis like Ryde's (1975), that is, communication occurring in a state of increased concentration and receptivity. The communication may include suggestions, and the change in receptivity be due to relaxation, trust in the therapist and/or some deeper change in arousal, such as a trance. Individual workers claim extremely high success rates for hypnosis, suggesting perhaps that if the therapist is good, and the client pays enough, it can work. However, while it remains a possibility that hypnosis, whatever it is, may suit some smokers, no controlled or comparative trials have shown it to be better than simple support plus a placebo (Raw, 1978).

ELECTRIC AVERSION THERAPY

Electric aversion therapy was very popular with psychologists for a while as a treatment for a variety of problems, including sexual disorders, alcoholism and smoking. It was popular because of theoretical appeal, having been derived directly from learning theory, and because it was so simple to apply (McGuire and Vallance, 1964). Smoking, for its part, would seem to be an ideal problem since it involves simple actions upon which the electric shock can be made contingent. As with hypnosis, however, the promise of early, uncontrolled trials was not maintained by later, more carefully controlled studies. In one such trial, Russell, Armstrong and Patel (1976) compared contingent shock, non-contingent shock, non-shock smoking (to control for the satiation effect), simple support, and no treatment. This last control group was not a waiting-list control. They were given a rationale for no treatment, namely that the assessment procedures showed that they did not need help and could stop smoking unaided, provided they made a firm decision to. All four treatments were effective in reducing or eliminating smoking and were superior to the control condition; 61% of the four treatment groups stopped smoking during the treatment period, compared with only 14% of the controls. There was no specific effect in favour of either contingent shock over non-contingent shock, or shock over simple support. Russell, Armstrong and Patel (1976) concluded: 'There is no evidence from this study that traditional conditioning processes play any part in the clinical response to electric aversion therapy. The clinical response to aversion therapy is non-specific and attributable to the host of other psychological factors and cognitive processes involved in clinical situations which influence and contribute to the therapeutic outcome of all psychological treatments.' They have not published follow-up results of this study.

SATIATION

Satiation involves increasing the rate of smoking until it becomes unpleasant, with the aim of eliminating the desire to smoke and creating revulsion at even the thought of a cigarette. In one study entitled 'A short duration group treatment of smoking behaviour by stimulus saturation' (Marrone, Merksamer and Salzberg, 1970) clients had to chain smoke (in a motel) for either 10 or 20 hours. A returnable cash deposit was used to ensure compliance with instructions. The results at 4 months follow-up showed an advantage for the 20-hour group (60% abstinent compared with 18% of the 10-hour group and 10% of untreated controls). However, this is a rather short period allowed for follow-up, and the method also seems somewhat impractical for normal clinical use. Evidence from the rapid smoking method does show, however, that over-smoking can eliminate the desire to smoke (Russell *et al.*, 1978).

RAPID SMOKING

Rapid smoking evolved from a conditioning paradigm in which hot smoky air rather than an electric shock was used as the aversive stimulus (Wilde, 1964). This was seen by Wilde as an attempt to produce an aversion to the taste of cigarette smoking using a 'natural' taste stimulus, cigarette smoke. He used a simple electric ventilator-heater to blow hot cigarette smoke into the face of a smoker contingent upon his smoking, or cool mentholated air contingent on stopping smoking. Although his short-term success rate was good (57%) there was no follow-up or control group, and he was suitably circumspect in his discussion.

Lichtenstein *et al.* (1973; Schmahl, Lichtenstein and Harris, 1972) investigated the use of warm smoky air and an increased smoking rate (rapid smoking), publishing two papers which promoted rapid smoking as a new, successful treatment. In the first study (Schmahl, Lichtenstein and Harris, 1972) two groups of smokers (seen individually) had to smoke rapidly, inhaling on command every 6 sec until they could tolerate no more. While thus smoking they received either hot smoky air blown in their faces or cool mentholated air. At the end of a trial clients would rest for a short time and then continue the procedure, until finally they could not tolerate another cigarette. The therapists had themselves stopped smoking by this method. Clients were strongly forbidden to smoke between sessions and were offered booster sessions at any hour of the night or day should the urge to smoke be too great. By the end of treatment all clients had stopped smoking. Clients were phoned monthly during follow-up for 6 months and at this time 57% were still abstinent. There were no differences in outcome between the two treatment groups, and the authors conceded that 'the data on treatment components are not clearly interpretable'.

In the second study (Lichtenstein *et al.*, 1973) smokers were assigned to four treatment conditions: warm smoky air plus rapid smoking, warm smoky air only, rapid smoking only (using the same procedure as in the first study), and an attention placebo procedure involving some normal smoking on command at the clinic, and lobeline pills between sessions. They were again followed up by monthly phone calls for 6 months; 98% stopped smoking during treatment and 53% were still abstinent at 6 months follow-up. During treatment there were no significant differences in outcome between any of the groups, but the relapse rate was higher for the attention placebo group, with 30% abstinent at 6 months follow-up compared with 60% in each of the three aversion groups. The resistance to relapse of the treatment group does suggest some sort of treatment effect, although not for rapid smoking compared with warm smoky air, and Lichtenstein *et al.* interpret it as an aversive effect.

A third study (Harris and Lichtenstein, 1971) gave all clients rapid smoking but varied three 'non-specific' social variables. Clients received either high or low social reinforcement during treatment along three dimensions: the therapist–client relationship, expectation of success, verbal reinforcement for abstinence. The manipulation produced a strong effect at the end of treatment and at 3 months follow-up, 72% of the 'high' group being abstinent at follow-up compared with 6% of the 'low' group (all the 'high' clients were abstinent at the end of treatment). Lichtenstein's group thus seem to be highly successful at stopping people smoking, but support for their rapid-smoking technique *per se* is weak.

Several other studies have failed to show rapid smoking to be better than other methods or controls, and most studies by other workers have achieved considerably lower success rates (Glasgow, 1979; Lando, 1975; Raw and Russell, 1980; Saterfield, 1977; Sutherland *et al.*, 1975). The evidence in favour of a clinically relevant specific effect of rapid smoking, therefore, is weak, although it does eliminate the desire to smoke (Raw and Russell, 1980) and may therefore be useful at the beginning of a more comprehensive stop-smoking programme. However, it does raise blood nicotine and carboxyhaemoglobin levels considerably (Russell *et al.*, 1978), and so should not be used with people suffering from cardiovascular disease.

COMPARATIVE TREATMENT TRIALS

There is no compelling evidence so far for the effectiveness of any specific treatment methods This is not to say that some methods are not better than others, but rather that they are not so much better that they warrant the time and energy needed to deliver them. The 20-hour satiation technique is a good example of this. Rapid smoking illustrates another important point. Until a new technique has been replicated by workers other than its progenitors it cannot truly be said to work. Subjected to this test, rapid smoking is found wanting. The evidence rather suggests that high short-term success rates can be achieved, but that they are probably due to 'non-specific' factors rather than to specific treatment techniques. These factors could be described as the motivation of the smokers (that is, no treatment will work if the smoker does not want to stop, but if she or he does, then any treatment will work), the structure offered/imposed by the clinic/treatment course and the support offered by the therapist (McFall and Hammen, 1971). These factors would account for what are sometimes called placebo effects, and it is obvious that in psychological treatments, as well as in many apparently physical treatments, the placebo response is very important.

A number of studies have compared different treatment methods, some of them using a control, and the results of these studies show the relative unimportance of specific treatment techniques compared with motivation and support. This conclusion is found in the following studies: Koenig and Masters (1965), who compared systematic desensitization, electric aversion, and attention placebo; Ober (1968) – operant self-control, self-administered electric aversion, transactional analysis; Keutzer (1968) – coverant control, breath-holding aversion, satiation, placebo drugs; Lawson and May (1970) – covert sensitization coverant control, contractual management, attention placebo; Bernstein (1970) – group therapy, attention placebo, told to stop using own efforts and given rationale for success; Marston and McFall (1971) – satiation, gradual reduction, aversive pill, support; Sipich, Russell and Tobias (1975) – covert sensitization, attention placebo, self-control; Wisocki and Rooney (1974) – thought stopping, covert sensitization, attention placebo.

The following studies achieved small specific effects which disappeared in the first few months of treatment, or small specific effects which were not significant statistically: Whitman (1969) – group discussion, self-administered electric aversion, operant self-control; Sachs, Bean and Morrow (1970) – covert sensitization, self-control, attention placebo; Wagner and Bragg (1970) – covert sensitization, systematic desensitization, both combined, relaxation, attention placebo; Sutherland *et al.* (1975) – satiation, relaxation, satiation plus relaxation.

Bernstein's (1970) thorough study in which he included only 'non-specific' treatments such as group discussion and support led him to conclude that some treatment was better than none but that it did not really matter what the treatment was. He named the non-specific components of therapy thus: 'participation in an experiment, expectation of change, suggestion, contact with an experimenter or leader and the like'. McFall and Hammen (1971) concurred, on the basis of their study which compared what they described as non-specific non-treatment: 'The outcome of the nontreatment clinic programme was comparable to others reviewed and suggests that the nonspecific factors studied may account for the temporary behaviour change found in most smoking treatment'. Actually their overall abstinence rates of 26% at the end of treatment and 5% at 6 months follow-up does not quite support their conclusion, so that other factors may have to be taken into account; for instance, perhaps the 'placebo' response to treatment depends on the amount of impressiveness of treatment, or the enthusiasm of the therapist. This is hardly an exceptional idea; in fact, it would be quite surprising if the therapist did not make any difference. Even this represents a problem though since the ideal 'treatment' is not only effective, but reliable, and is effective in the hands of different therapists. Finally, it is also cost-effective. It is doubtful whether the stop-smoking treatment reviewed so far could satisfy all these criteria and the search for a cost-effective treatment may prove more fruitful than the search for an effective treatment. Such considerations, as well as the logical one of looking for a pharmacological solution to a problem acknowledged to have a pharmacological component, led to the development and testing of a genuine nicotine substitute: nicotine chewing gum.

NICOTINE CHEWING GUM

Nicotine chewing gum (Nicorette) was developed and is manufactured by a Swedish pharmaceutical company, Leo of Helsingborg. It is available in two strengths: 2 mg or 4 mg of nicotine to each piece of gum, although most clinical trials have used the 2 mg gum. The stronger gum seems to be too strong for most smokers. The nicotine is bound to an ion exchange resin which allows it to be released slowly as the gum is chewed. The gum is also buffered to a pH of about 8.5 to promote absorption of the nicotine through the buccal mucosa, since any nicotine that is swallowed is largely wasted (Russell and Feyerabend, 1978). The rate of absorption of nicotine from the gum depends on the vigour and rate of chewing. The 2 mg gum produces nicotine levels in the blood of about half those achieved by normal smoking, but this appears to satisfy clients who are trying to stop smoking (Raw *et al.*, 1980). Clinical results with the gum are promising so far (Russell, Raw and Jarvis, 1980). In an uncontrolled trial, which was designed to achieve as high a success rate as possible, and did not use a placebo comparison, a 1 year success rate of 38% has been achieved (Raw *et al.*, 1980). Each claim of abstinence was validated by measurement of expired air carbon monoxide (Jarvis, Russell and Saloojee, 1980). The 69 people in this study chewed an average of eight pieces of 2 mg Nicorette per day for the first few months and only six people (9%) chewed it for more than a year. Of these six only two were still chewing the gum at 2 years. In view of the fact that these were heavy (32 cigarettes per day compared with the national average of 18) and dependent (they needed to come to a clinic) smokers, this figure is both surprisingly low, and extremely encouraging. Only 13% of these people complained of side-effects from the gum and in only two cases were these unpleasant enough for the people concerned to stop using the gum.

Few double-blind controlled trials have been published yet with Nicorette, but the results of studies completed so far are promising. Puska, Bjorkqvist and Koskela, (1979) found the gum to be better than placebo at the end of treatment (success rates of 70 versus 54%) but not at 6 months follow-up (35% versus 28%). Fagerstrom (1981) on the other hand found Nicorette to be significantly better than placebo at 6 months follow-up (63% versus 45%) and Fee and Stewart (1981) found it to be better than placebo at the end of treatment (46% versus 33%). Although the success rates vary they are quite high compared with purely psychological methods, so that nicotine chewing gum may turn out to be effective as well as cost-effective. It has the obvious advantage that it can be prescribed by doctors, which means that through general practitioners it can reach most smokers, and this is something which has never before been true of any treatment method. However it is not a panacea. Results with the gum show that smokers need time to get used to it, and tend to dislike its taste at first. This means that they need careful and patient training in how to use the gum, and it is possible that success rates will go down when the gum is not used by experienced therapists. The corollary of this is that doctors will have to be trained how to use the gum properly. Although the gum looks extremely promising, presumably because it does something to alleviate the withdrawal pangs, stopping smoking remains a lengthy and difficult process which requires the smoker's patience and determination. If the gum is given to smokers carelessly, with little instruction or follow-up, it could be ineffective, and it is important to investigate its effectiveness in the hands of doctors. Two such trials, one with chest physicians and one with several practitioners, are already in progress in Britain in 1981.

THE ROLE OF DOCTORS

The real significance of nicotine chewing gum does not lie in its success rate, although that is encouraging. Even with a 100% success rate it would take the clinics in Britain 1500 years to help all the current smokers to stop smoking, and there is no likelihood of the number of clinics increasing substantially. Clearly no treatment method can solve the smoking problem. The advantage of nicotine chewing gum lies in the fact that it can be prescribed by doctors. There are more than 20 000 general practitioners in Britain at the moment, so that with even a modest success rate they could help many thousands of smokers stop, and I have already discussed the evidence that there is real demand for help in stopping. It has been shown that with simple but firm advice to stop smoking, plus a leaflet and the warning of follow-up, general practitioners can help about 5% of their patients stop smoking (Russell *et al.*, 1979). This alone would yield more than 500 000 ex-smokers in Britain now, though presumably, after a few years when the less dependent smokers had stopped, the yield would go down. Nicotine chewing gum however could be expected to increase it, and give general practitioners a way of helping smokers who at present need the support and specialist help of clinics.

THE POTENTIAL ROLE OF THE MASS MEDIA

The mass media have not yet been used in Britain in a serious attempt to help people stop smoking. There is therefore little evidence as to their potential effectiveness. A recent follow-up of the effects of a brief television programme about stopping smoking showed a rather disappointing success rate, at 1 year follow-up, of 1% of those who cooperated in the study. Since these were only 12% of the sample contacted, the results are extremely poor. However, the programme, which was broadcast to an estimated five million people, did draw a response from about 500 000 people who took the trouble to phone or write, asking for an antismoking kit (Raw and van der Pligt, 1981). Clearly then there are millions of smokers who feel they need help in stopping smoking, who could be reached by television and the medium has yet to be tested properly in this role.

GRADUAL OR SUDDEN STOPPING?

Advice on whether smokers should try to cut down gradually, or stop suddenly, varies from expert to expert, from booklet to booklet, with rarely any justification offered for the advice given. Smokers often feel it would be better to cut down gradually not because they feel it would be the better way but because they are afraid of stopping and want to put off the day – in which case gradual reduction probably will not help, since it is rather beside the point. There is little good research evidence upon which to decide the issue. Most treatment studies emphasize the need for clients to stop straight away, and some published studies show that those who succeed in stopping in the longer term, stop within the first few days of treatment (Raw and Russell, 1980). The self-control studies, on the other hand, stress gradual reduction in the context of gradually reshaping one's habit patterns and, on the whole, their results are worse than those of the other treatment studies. In Bernard and Efran's (1972) gradual reduction study it is interesting that in spite of instructions to cut down gradually, the successful clients had stopped outright. If this clue is valid then it may be that gradual reduction is inherently more difficult than sudden stopping. A finding which may be relevant to this issue is reported by Shiffman and Jarvik (1976) who observed that smokers who stopped outright reported less severe craving in the first 2 weeks of abstinence than smokers who only cut down. It may be that intermittent smoking while ultimately trying to stop undermines motivation to stop, perhaps by increasing enjoyment of the few cigarettes. At the very least it means continuation of the habit so that it is already available, as it were, when stress comes along to precipitate relapse. Much of this is speculation, however, and requires further research. On the basis of both the evidence available and on my own clinical experience, smokers should be advised to make a clean break and stop suddenly.

LOW TAR CIGARETTES

Somehow the tobacco companies have persuaded many smokers that low tar cigarettes are less dangerous than higher tar cigarettes. Presumably this is partly because smokers want to believe this and it seems a commonly held belief that low tar cigarettes are 'OK' or 'relatively safe'. However, there are few grounds for this belief. Evidence already discussed on the role of nicotine in smoking, and especially showing the lack of relationship between the nicotine yield of cigarettes and blood nicotine levels (Russell *et al.*, 1980), suggests that smokers regulate their smoking to maintain an optimal blood nicotine level. This means that if smokers switch to a lower nicotine cigarette which, since tar and nicotine levels are so highly correlated means low tar as well, they will inhale more smoke in order to maintain the same dose of nicotine, in which case they could even absorb more tar and carbon monoxide, not less. There is evidence for such compensatory inhaling (Russell *et al.*, 1978), so that many smokers who make this switch are certainly no safer. This needs to be explained to smokers so that they can either (if they really cannot stop) switch to a cigarette that has a better tar:nicotine *ratio* (a medium nicotine:low tar cigarette would be better) or stop deceiving themselves.

The same principle applies to cutting down. Up to a point, reduced consumption, measured in cigarettes per day, can be compensated for by increased inhalation, so that cutting down from 80 to 20 a day could be useless from a health point of view. One smoker attending the Maudsley Smokers Clinic did this, and was very proud of his achievement. But his carboxyhaemoglobin level at 6 months follow-up was the same as it had been when he first attended the clinic, indicating that he was effectively still smoking the same.

Finally, the same principle applies to switching to a pipe or cigars. There is no point in making this switch, since the likelihood is that the smoker will continue inhaling (Turner, Sillett and McNicol, 1981). The relative safety of pipe and cigar smokers is almost certainly based on the fact that most primary (that is, who have never been cigarette smokers) pipe or cigar smokers do not inhale. Again, a smoker from the Maudsley Smokers Clinic gave up cigarettes and switched to a pipe, believing that he was not inhaling. However his carboxyhaemoglobin level was 6.0%, indicating fairly heavy inhalation.

Logically, the only way to avoid the risks attached to smoking is to stop. However some smokers find this too difficult and, as we have seen, it is no good them switching to a pipe or cigars or cutting down. If smokers do smoke for nicotine but die from tar, they need to get the nicotine in a way which does not also deliver tar. They could chew nicotine chewing gum, though this seems unlikely to catch on, partly because chewing is also considered a nasty habit in Britain, and partly because it does not taste very pleasant. Nor does it deliver nicotine in as satisfying a way as cigarettes do. They could chew tobacco though this seems as unlikely to become popular. The final choice seems to be to return to snuff, which has been shown to produce a fairly quick rate of absorption of nicotine (Russell, Jarvis and Feyerabend, 1980), and so might be an acceptable alternative for cigarette smokers who cannot stop.

DISCUSSION

Progress in helping people stop smoking has been slow, and the slow but steady fall in the prevalence of smoking since about 1973 cannot be attributed to it. Smoking clinics play, and have always played a peripheral role. There has never been any integrated policy on smoking into which clinics can fit, and consequently clinics have only sprung up where there have been workers interested and committed enough to run them. They have often been run by people with little access to research findings and no prior experience of either smoking or group work. Consequently many clinics have had discouraging results, which in turn has led 'experts' and health administrators to question their usefulness. In fact the usefulness of clinics as part of an overall antismoking strategy has not been fairly tested, and will not have been until there are more better run and well-publicized clinics. Their role then would be to help to stop smoking those smokers who want to stop but are too dependent (for whatever reason) to do so unaided. We do not know how many such smokers there are, but the well-run and well-known clinics that already exist are very busy, and there is no doubt that there is a demand for help. However, clinics could probably not satisfy this demand entirely, and their other important role is to act as advice and resource centres for their communities. They could do this partly by offering people help to start groups and partly through literature designed to help individuals and groups help themselves stop smoking.

Part of the problem facing clinics has been the lack of effective methods, and low success rates have undoubtedly led to low attendance at clinics, subsequent loss of interest or morale by staff and closing of clinics. The psychological research has offered little hope of a breakthrough and where clinics have survived, it has usually been because of the energy and dedication of its workers, not because of its success. The advent of nicotine chewing gum is therefore important. It represents the first genuine breakthrough in smoking withdrawal treatment, in both effectiveness and practicality. It seems to have increased the success rate dramatically at the Maudsley Smokers Clinic (Raw *et al.*, 1980), and it is relatively easy and non-time-consuming to administer. It could improve clinic success rates and consequently morale, throughput and visibility in their communities. More importantly, the gum can be prescribed by doctors and so provides for the first time a real incentive for general practitioners to become involved in helping people stop smoking. It is important though that the gum is not thought of as a cure in itself. The most important aspect of stopping smoking is still motivation, and the gum should not be given to people who are not fairly strongly motivated to stop smoking. Ideally then, doctors prescribing the gum should also offer follow-up appointments, so that the smoker also feels supported psychologically. If the smoker is very dependent and needs regular support she or he should be referred to a clinic or group. It is at this stage, of course, that the ideal breaks down. Investigation of the potential role of health education departments is required to see if they could cooperate with group practices and health centres in providing help for smokers. Some of this research is under way.

There remains a need for urgent action from the government. Most smoking experts agree that cigarettes should be more expensive, a policy which would deter smokers (Russell, 1973) *and* increase tax revenue. Even at 1980 prices (roughly 75 pence for 20 cigarettes) cigarettes were nearly half their 1950 price compared with average disposable income. Even more urgent is the need for legislation on the advertising and promotion of tobacco products, which must at least contribute to the 'adult', sophisticated image of smoking, which in turn must account for its attractiveness to children. Preventing children smoking is obviously the most important priority for reducing smoking-related diseases in the future, and our almost total ignorance of why children smoke and how to prevent them is both astonishing and dismaying. However that goal cannot be pursued in isolation from reducing smoking in adults, since children will presumably continue to smoke while adult models exist. Again an integrated policy is needed, but the government should accept responsibility for funding more research on smoking and children, and for seeing that children cannot get hold of cigarettes, nor be exposed to images of smoking projected by advertising. Efforts in this direction so far can only be described as token.

Reasons for lack of government action are not hard to find. The conflict of interests is rather obvious, but it is essentially financial and it is rather depressing that no government has yet considered its moral responsibility on the issue, nor even its duty to respond to changing social attitudes towards smoking. Meanwhile it is important to continue trying to persuade and help people to stop smoking, and the final section considers practical ways in which this can be done now.

HOW TO HELP SMOKERS STOP

A small, pocket-sized booklet which gives simple but detailed advice on how to stop smoking is currently available from the author (Raw, 1980). It is entitled *How to Stop Smoking*, and describes a straightforward plan of action based on the author's experience of helping people stop smoking at the Maudsley Smokers Clinic. The *Readers Digest* will soon be publishing a Family Medical Adviser which will contain a short section entitled 'Smoking: the risks and how to stop' (Raw, 1982). This section includes a careful restating of the risks of smoking, with an explanation of why the evidence is so strong, as well as a 'how to stop' plan. If there is sufficient demand copies of this feature will be made available as a leaflet for clinicians to give to smokers. Publication is expected some time in 1982. Finally, the following simple guide could be used by a busy clinician who can spare a few minutes to advise someone to stop smoking:

(1) Find out about the patient's attitude towards stopping smoking (that is, assess motivation).
(2) Advise the patient firmly to stop smoking; add all relevant motivating information.
(3) Give basic guidance on how to stop.
(4) Offer as much support as seems necessary, or is possible; preferably offer at least one follow-up appointment.
(5) Be firm but sympathetic.

The doctor should first discover whether the patient wants to stop and/or believes smoking to be harmful to him or her personally. The doctor should then supply any relevant motivating information and strongly advise the patient to stop smoking. At this stage he must assess whether it is worth saying or doing anything more. If the patient does not really want to stop smoking, there is little he can do. If the patient seems receptive he can offer the following basic principles which should be backed up, at the very least, with the *How to Stop Smoking* booklet, which follows the same plan:

(1) Be sure you want to stop.
(2) Be sure of your reasons.
(3) Set a D-day for stopping that suits you, but is within a week or two from now.
(4) Stop on that day. Do not try to cut down gradually beforehand.
(5) Ask your friends not to offer you cigarettes.
(6) If you cannot help smoking when drinking, avoid pubs and alcohol for the first few weeks.
(7) Do not relax your vigilance for at least 6 months, though the worst of the withdrawal should be over within 4–6 weeks.
(8) Work out in advance how you are going to cope with problems and/or crises, especially tension, loss of concentration and other people offering you cigarettes.
(9) Do not be tempted to try tranquillizers, as they will not help.
(10) Save the money you would have spent on cigarettes and treat yourself.

Ideally the doctor should offer a follow-up appointment in about 1, 3 and 6 months time and if possible, and the patient needs it, arrange follow-up and support through some other agency, possibly community nurses, health education officers or the local clinic if there is one. An up-to-date list of all smoking withdrawal clinics in England and Wales is always available from ASH. Finally, if the patient is *very* dependent (smokes heavily, which could mean anything over 20 cigarettes per day, inhales deeply, and has tried and failed to stop before, succeeding for shorter and shorter periods), prescribe nicotine chewing gum (Nicorette), details of which can be found in Raw *et al.* (1980) and Russell, Raw and Jarvis (1980).

ACKNOWLEDGEMENTS

I would like to thank Julia Heller for helpful comments on a draft of this paper.

REFERENCES

Bartlett, W. A. and Whitehead, R. W. (1957). The effectiveness of meprobamate and lobeline as smoking deterrents. *J. Lab. Clin. Med.*, **50**, 278

Bergler, E. (1946). Psychopathology of compulsive smoking. *Psychiatr. Q.*, **20**, 297

Bernard, H. S. and Efran, J. S. (1972). Eliminating versus reducing smoking using pocket timers. *Behav. Res. Ther.*, **10**, 399

Bernstein, D. A. (1970). The modification of smoking behaviour: a search for effective variables. *Behav. Res. Ther.*, **8**, 133

Bewley, B. R., Day, I. and Ide, L. (1973). *Smoking by Children in Great Britain.* London: SSRC/MRC

Bewley, B., Johnson, M., Bland, J. and Murray, M. (1980). Trends in children's smoking. *Commun. Med.*, **2**, 186

Blumberg, H. H., Cohen, S. D., Dronfield, B. E., Mordecai, E. A., Roberts, J. C. and Hawks, D. (1974). British opiate users: 1. People approaching London drug treatment centres. *Int. J. Addict.*, **9**, 1

Bynner, J. M. (1969). *The Young Smoker.* London: HMSO

Capell, P. J. (1978). Trends in cigarette smoking in the United Kingdom. *Health Trends.* London: Department of Health and Social Security

Davison, G. C. and Rosen, R. C. (1972). Lobeline and reduction of cigarette smoking. *Psychol. Rep.*, **31**, 443

Dorsey, J. L. (1936). Control of the tobacco habit. *Ann. Intern. Med.*, **10**, 628

Edwards, G. (1964). Double blind trial of lobeline in an anti-smoking clinic. *Med. Off.*, **112**, 158

Ejrup, B. (1964). Treatment of tobacco addiction: experiences in tobacco withdrawal clinics; can we help them stop? *Am. Cancer Soc.* Chicago

Fagerstrom, Karl-Olov (1981). A comparison of psychological and pharmacological treatment in smoking cessation. *Lakartidningen*, **78**, 1082

Fee, W. M. and Stewart, M. J. (1981). A controlled trial of nicotine chewing gum in a smoking withdrawal clinic. *Practitioner*, **226**, 148

Ford, S. and Ederer, F. (1965). Breaking the cigarette habit. *J. Am. Med. Assoc.*, **194**, 119

Glasgow, R. E. (1979). The effects of a self-control manual and amount of therapist contact in the modification of smoking behaviour, unpublished PhD thesis, University of Oregon

Harris, D. E. and Lichtenstein, E. (1971). The contribution of nonspecific social variables to a successful behavioral treatment of smoking. Paper read to Western Psychological Association, USA

Ingersoll, W. and Sekonda, W. (1981). Gradual reduction of smoking by a timing device. *Watchtower Rev.*, **60**, 1

Jarvis, M., Russell, M. A. H. and Saloojee, Y. (1980). Expired air carbon monoxide: a simple breath test of tobacco smoke intake. *Br. Med. J.*, **281**, 484

Johnson, E. and Donoghue, J. R. (1971). Hypnosis and smoking: a review of the literature. *Am. J. Clin. Hypnosis*, **13**, 265

Keutzer, C. S. (1968). Behaviour modification of smoking: the experimental investigation of diverse techniques, *Behav. Res. Ther.*, **6**, 137

Koenig, K. P. and Masters, J. (1965). Experimental treatment of habitual smoking. *Behav. Res. Ther.*, **3**, 235

Lando, H. A. (1975). A comparison of excessive and rapid smoking in the modification of chronic smoking behaviour. *J. Consulting Clin. Psychol.*, **43**, 350

Lawson, D. M. and May, R. B. (1970). Three procedures for the extinction of smoking behaviour. *Psychol. Rec.*, **20**, 151

Lichtenstein, E., Harris, D. E., Birchler, G. R., Wahl, J. M. and Schmahl, D. P. (1973). Comparison of rapid smoking, warm smoky air, and attention placebo in the modification of smoking behaviour. *J. Consulting Clin. Psychol.*, **40**, 92

Marrone, R. L., Merksamer, M. A. and Salzberg, P. M. (1970). A short duration group treatment of smoking behaviour by stimulus saturation. *Behav. Res. Ther.*, **8**, 347

Marston, A. R. and McFall, R. M. (1971). Comparison of behaviour modification approaches to smoking reduction. *J. Consulting Clin. Psychol.*, **36**, 153

McFall, R. M. and Hammen, C. L. (1971). Motivation, structure and self-monitoring: role of nonspecific factors in smoking reduction. *J. Consulting Clin. Psychol.*, **37**, 80

McFarland, J. W., Gimbel, H. W., Donald, W. A. J., Folkenberg, E. J. (1964). The 5-day programme to help individuals stop smoking. *Connecticut Med.*, **28**, 885

McGuire, R. J. and Vallance, M. (1964). Aversion therapy by electric shock: a simple technique. *Br. Med. J.*, **1**, 151

McKennell, A. C. and Thomas, R. K. (1967). *Adults and Adolescents: Smoking Habits and Attitudes*. London: HMSO

Merry, J. and Preston, G. (1963). The effect of buffered lobeline sulphate on cigarette smoking. *Practitioner*, **190**, 628

Ober, D. C. (1968). Modification of smoking behaviour. *J. Consulting Clin. Psychol.*, **32**, 543

Office of Population Censuses and Surveys (1978). *General Household Survey*, pp. 127–133, London: HMSO

Puska, P., Bjorkqvist, S. and Koskela, K. (1979). Nicotine-containing chewing gum in smoking cessation: a double-blind trial with half year follow-up. *Addictive Behav.*, **4**, 141

Raw, M. (1978). The treatment of cigarette dependence. In Y. Israel *et al.* (eds.) *Research Advances in Alcohol and Drug Problems*, Chapter 11, vol. 4. New York: Plenum

Raw, M. (1980). *How to Stop Smoking*. London: ASH

Raw, M. (1982). Smoking: the risks and how to stop. *Readers Digest Family Medical Adviser*

Raw, M., Jarvis, M. J., Feyerabend, C. and Russell, M. A. H. (1980). Comparison of nicotine chewing gum and psychological treatments for dependent smokers. *Br. Med. J.*, **281**, 481

Raw, M. and Russell, M. A. H. (1980). Rapid smoking, cue exposure and support in the modification of smoking. *Behav. Res. Ther.*, **18**, 363
Raw, M. and van der Pligt, J. (1981). *Can Television Help People Stop Smoking. Health Education and the Media.* Oxford: Pergamon
Ross, C. A. (1967). Smoking withdrawal research clinics. *Am. J. Public Health*, **57**, 677
Russell, M. A. H. (1973). Changes in cigarette price and consumption by men in Britain 1946–71. *Br. J. Prevent Social Med.*, **27**, 1
Russell, M. A. H. (1976). Tobacco smoking and nicotine dependence. In R. J. Gibbins *et al.* (eds.) *Research Advances in Alcohol and Drug Problems.* Vol. 3. New York: John Wiley
Russell, M. A. H. (1980). Nicotine intake and its regulation. *J. Psychosomatic Res.*, **24**, 253
Russell, M. A. H., Armstrong, E. and Patel, U. A. (1976). Temporal contiguity in electric aversion therapy for cigarette smoking. *Behav. Res. Ther.*, **14**, 103
Russell, M. A. H. and Feyerabend, C. (1978). Cigarette smoking: a dependence on high nicotine boli. *Drug Metabol. Rev.*, **8**, 29
Russell, M. A. H., Jarvis, M., Iyer, R. and Feyerabend, C. (1980). Relation of nicotine yield of cigarettes to blood nicotine concentrations in smokers. *Br. Med. J.*, **280**, 972
Russell, M. A. H., Jarvis, M. J. and Feyerabend, C. (1980). A new age for snuff? *Lancet*, **1**, 474
Russell, M. A. H., Raw, M. and Jarvis, M. J. (1980). The clinical use of nicotine chewing gum. *Br. Med. J.*, **1**, 1599
Russell, M. A. H., Raw, M., Taylor, C., Feyerabend, C. and Saloojee, Y. (1978). Blood nicotine and carboxyhaemoglobin levels after rapid smoking aversion therapy. *J. Consulting Clin. Psychol.*, **46**, 1423
Russell, M. A. H., Sutton, S. R., Feyerabend, C. and Cole, P. V. (1978). Addiction Research Unit nicotine litration studies. In R. E. Thornton (ed.). *Smoking Behaviour. Physiological and Psychological Influences.* Edinburgh: Churchill Livingstone
Russell, M. A. H., Wilson, C., Taylor, C. and Baker, C. D. (1979). Effect of general practitioner's advice against smoking. *Br. Med. J.*, **2**, 231
Ryde, D. (1975). On hypnosis. *Med. News*, **June 19**
Sachs, L. B., Bean, H. and Morrow, J. E. (1970). Comparison of smoking treatments. *Behav. Ther.*, **1**, 465
Saterfield, H. D. (1977). Efficacy of self-destruction as a treatment component in smoking cessation. Unpublished PhD thesis, Stanford University
Schmahl, D., Lichtenstein, E. and Harris, D. E. (1972). Successful treatment of habitual smokers with warm smoky air and rapid smoking. *J. Consulting Clin. Psychol.*, **36**, 105
Schwartz, J. L. and Dubitzky, M. (1968). One year follow-up results of a smoking cessation program. *Can. J. Public Health*, **59**, 161
Shiffman, S. M. and Jarvik, M. E. (1976). Smoking withdrawal symptoms in two weeks of abstinence. *Psychopharmacology*, **50**, 35
Sipich, J. F., Russell, R. K. and Tobias, L. L. (1975). A comparison of covert sensitization and 'nonspecific' treatment in the modification of smoking behaviour. *J. Behav. Ther. Exper. Psychiatry*, **5**, 201
Stepney, R. (1980). Smoking behaviour: a psychology of the cigarette habit. *Br. J. Chest Dis.*, **74**, 325
Sutherland, A., Amit, Z., Golden, M. and Roseberger, Z. (1975). Comparison of three behavioural techniques in the modification of smoking behaviour. *J. Consulting Clin. Psychol.*, **43**, 443

Turle, G. C. (1958). An investigation into the therapeutic action of hydroxyzine (Atarax) in the treatment of nervous disorders and the control of the tobacco habit. *J. Mental Sci.*, **104**, 826
Turner, J. A. M., Sillett, R. W. and McNicol, M. W. (1981). The inhaling habits of pipe smokers. *Br. J. Chest Dis.*, **75**, 71
Wagner, M. K. and Bragg, R. A. (1970). Comparing behavior modification approaches to habit decrement-smoking. *J. Consulting Clin. Psychol.*, **34**, 258
Wald, N. (1978). Smoking as a cause of disease. In A. E. Bennett (ed.) *Recent Advances in Community Medicine*. Edinburgh: Churchill Livingstone
Whitehead, R. W. and Davies, J. M. A. (1964). A study of methylphenidate and diazepam as possible smoking deterrents. *Curr. Ther. Res. Clin. Exp.*, **6**, 363
Whitman, T. L. (1969). Modification of chronic smoking behaviour: a comparison of three approaches. *Behav. Res. Ther.*, **7**, 257
Wilde, G. J. S. (1964). Behaviour therapy for addicted cigarette smokers. *Behav. Res. Ther.*, **2**, 107
Wisocki, P. A. and Rooney, E. J. (1974). A comparison of thought stopping and covert sensitization techniques in the treatment of smoking: a brief report. *Psychol. Rec.*, **24**, 191

9

Compulsive overeating

J. Hubert Lacey

The most noteworthy aspect of compulsive overeating is that the majority of complainants are women. An attempt to understand the disorders associated with compulsive eating must focus on this observation and explain it. The very fact that there is such a profound discrepancy in this behaviour between the sexes suggests that the pathology is rooted in sexuality. This is not to imply that the problem is one of sexual dysfunction (and associated with the act of intercourse) but rather related to those concepts which differentiate masculinity and femininity.

Superficially, what marks out an adult woman from a man is her size and shape, the differences in shape being composed, in the main, of fat tissue. Women are more fatty than men; a healthy man has about 14% of his body weight in the form of storage fat tissue, and a woman has about 18%.

This relationship between fat and female sexuality is emphasized by the timing in a woman's life when fat is deposited, the sites of those deposits and their function.

The first rapid increase in fat deposition occurs at puberty. Further fat deposition occurs during pregnancy and sometimes at the menopause: all events which are sexually determined. In the pubescent girl, first sexual emotions are associated with, and emphasized by, a dramatic change in shape and weight, and by menstruation. These events declare to the girl, her family and her peers that she is preparing, psychologically and physiologically, for reproduction. They draw attention to the changing nature of relationships both within and outside the family, and for the need for new social skills about which she feels unsure.

The profound changes in female body shape are the result of a general increase in subcutaneous fat, together with concentrations of fat tissues at specific sites, especially the thighs, the breasts and the buttocks. Gluteal fat deposits are further emphasized in pubescence as the bony pelvis grows and the transverse diameter increases. Such deposits tend to delineate the female from the male, and hence have developed secondary sexual significance.

That women are fattier than men begs the question: why? Any answer is likely to remain contentious. Fat is mostly used in the body as a storage tissue of high energy. Could it be that such fat deposits in women provide, in evolutionary terms, a reservoir of sufficient energy to maintain pregnancy and lactation in the face of erratic food supplies? This view is reinforced by the findings that fat tissue mass and body weight appear to act as triggers for the pubertal process itself.

Two threshold weights have, so far, been delineated. Luteinizing hormone (LH) and follicle stimulating hormone (FSH) appear to be unresponsive to their releasing factors below a body weight of 43 kg. Work, with an anorexia nervosa population, refeeding in hospital, suggests that a mean body weight of 43 kg is necessary to trigger sexual hormone activity with its attendant feminization and psychological sexuality (Palmer *et al.*, 1975).

A second, similar but higher body weight threshold has been suggested, though this is more contentious. Rose Frisch (Frisch and McArthur, 1974), examining a general population of adolescent girls, has determined that menstruation occurs at a mean weight of 48 kg ($\pm$ 3.7 kg) and when at least 17% of body weight is in the form of fat tissue. These two distinct weight thresholds seem to initiate and complete the hormonal process of changing a girl into a woman. Body weight and fat tissue provide the driving force for this biological and psychological change. Given this, it is perhaps unsurprising that within the turmoil of pubertal change, dieting and bulimia (overeating) are widespread amongst teenage schoolgirls because, consciously or unconsciously, the association between their new uncertainty and their weight is recognized.

COMPULSIVE EATING IN GENERAL POPULATIONS

This pattern was shown in a recent study of the eating habits of 16–17-year-old-schoolgirls (Lacey *et al.*, 1978). The study demonstrated that eating behaviour, previously considered to be unusual or abnormal, was widespread. The girls demonstrated two distinct patterns of energy intake, each with its own periodicity. The first cycle was short and varied markedly day to day, with a tendency to be more pronounced towards the weekend. The mean daily variation of calorific intake was four-fold. (The range, however, was massive: one subject varied her intake by a factor of 10!) These daily swings were superimposed on a further cycle with a periodicity of about a month, energy intake tending to increase prior to menstruation and to decline immediately after it. This energy fluctuation was, in the main, secondary to carbohydrate manipulation, protein and fat intake tending to remain more stable. The study showed that periods of carbohydrate abstention or avoidance closely followed by bulimia, again particularly with carbohydrate foods, was a feature exhibited by all the girls. A binge with carbohydrate food is partially due to its easy availability. However, there may be a more deepseated reason. During man's evolution foods high in carbohydrate have tended to be the easiest for him to gather. Hence, they would have formed the basis of the energy needed to maintain the fat deposits whose procreative importance have been outlined above.

Compulsive overeating and 'dieting' are usually inseparable. This pattern of dietary manipulation is, in its milder form, ubiquitous in young female populations. The behaviour seems to be associated with the perception these young girls have of their bodies, and the socio-cultural factors which have influenced them.

Overperception of body shape, previously thought to be a hallmark of anorexia nervosa, is very common amongst all teenage girls. Thighs are particularly overperceived, and the erroneous body shape generally held is reminiscent of the exaggerated female form of a fertility goddess – a collective unconscious indeed! Unlike boys, who perceive their bodies as a whole, girls perceive their bodies part by part, and attempt to deal with any area which gives them dissatisfaction by general dieting (and consequent manipulation) (Crisp and Kalucy, 1974; Lacey *et al.*, 1975).

A study examining the total teenage population of a small Swedish town (Nylander, 1971) revealed that many girls thought themselves fat and that this feeling became common with increasing adolescent age, being reported by only 26% of the 14-year-olds, but by over half of the 18-year-olds in the sample. The investigation was conducted primarily by questionnaire under supervision. A further study (Huenemann *et al.*, 1966) looked at approximately 1000 teenagers in the American Public High School system. This study used anthropometric data as well as several questionnaires. The results revealed that teenagers have a great interest in body confirmation. The girls were particularly preoccupied with their shape and weight. About 50% of the girls classified themselves as obese, whereas only 25% of them were identified as obese in anthropometric terms.

In the Swedish study (Nylander, 1971), about one-third of the girls reported serious dietary manipulation. Such manipulation was more frequent among the older teenage girls and, not surprisingly, among those whose weight was above average. A substantial proportion of all girls reported that they had developed symptoms which were connected with their dietary manipulations. Thus, 10% of the sample described amenorrhoea and increased interest in food and food preparation within the context of compulsive eating or food avoidance. From Canada it has been reported that in a middle-class suburban population 5% of women vomited periodically as a means of controlling body weight. The apparent increase in this behaviour and feeling have been paralleled by the aesthetic preference of our culture for thinness in women. There is increased emphasis for women to appear slim, to diet and to exercise

(Gardner and Garfinkel, 1980). Further, manipulation of diet is more common in those subcultures in which there is excess pressure to be slim, such as ballet dancers and models.

Thus, severe dietary restriction, bulimia, psychogenic vomiting, overestimation of body shape and undue preoccupation with body weight are widespread features in general female populations.

THE BULIMIC SYNDROME

The degree of overeating necessary to cause distress varies wildly and depends more on individual response than on the amount of food consumed. Like most neurotic symptomatology, it arises as a response to difficulty or stress, especially of an interpersonal nature. Compulsive overeating can be experienced to an exaggerated degree, such that it becomes all-encompassing and life-disrupting.

When at this extreme of neurotic intensity the symptom can become the central pillar around which other dietary symptoms cluster, thereby forming a syndrome. This syndrome, occurring at normal body weight, is separated by definition from anorexia nervosa and massive obesity, and by degree from the mild periodic overeating which is so common in general female populations described above.

In recent years, this disorder, characterized by gorging and variously termed, has attracted increasing clinical attention. It has been called bulimorexia (Boskind-Lodahl, 1976), the dietary chaos syndrome (Palmer, 1979), bulimia nervosa (Russell, 1979), dysorexia (Vandereycken and Pierloot, 1980), hyperexia nervosa (Ziolko, 1976), and the thin–fat syndrome (Bruch, 1974). Within the diversity of symptoms offered by such patients it would be surprising if the clinical descriptions were identical; emphasis varies, which perhaps indicates the heterogeneous nature of the condition in both its clinical presentation and its aetiology. Some authors describe a comparatively mild condition; others a severe, crippling disorder, refractory to treatment. Some leave it undifferentiated from the bulimic form of anorexia nervosa, while others see it as an occasional sequela of anorectics after restoration of normal body weight.

While this author recognizes these conditions, the majority of patients complaining of bulimic symptoms give no such history. The bulimic syndrome is a disorder with a distinct clinical presentation and aetiological factors.

Patients with the bulimic syndrome present with normal, or near normal, body weight for age and height. There is no history of weight phobia, anorexia nervosa or major weight loss. Such a syndrome is quite distinct from anorexia nervosa, though related, for such patients do not show the phobia of normal body weight which is the pathognomonic feature of anorexia nervosa (Crisp, 1967). Neither do the patients demonstrate the essential features of anorexia nervosa as determined by Russell (1970). There is no morbid fear of becoming fat, although they do declare the normal female preoccupation with shape and weight

(Nylander, 1971) as described above. Their eating behaviour, though similar to the bulimic anorectic, does not lead to marked loss of body weight and malnutrition. Further, such patients do not fit the criteria established by Feighner (1972) as being necessary for the diagnosis of anorexia nervosa. These patients give no history of massive obesity and their body weight, though fluctuating, does not demonstrate the extreme fluctuations of the massively obese.

On presentation, the patient's initial complaint is of a turbulent pattern of eating, which by definition includes bulimia, and often self-induced vomiting and laxative abuse (Lacey, 1980). The bulimia is periodic, but chronic, and is associated with profound distress. There is a particular tendency to abuse carbohydrates or foods which the patient views as 'junk', or as lacking worth. Normal eating rarely occurs between the bulimic episodes, but rather the intervals are marked by abstinence or, more usually, forbearance of those particular foods which will later be wolfishly overindulged.

The patients are fascinated and haunted by *food*, particularly carbohydrate. Some use it in excess, as a sedative to calm the sense of chaos they feel in and around their lives, such that it develops an addictive quality. Others use it to cheapen and degrade themselves, an affront associated with guilt and secrecy. In addition, they feel that their eating pattern is *out of control*. This lack of control may extend to the abuse of alcohol or other drugs, and also to other appetites, particularly their sexual drives. They declare marked unsureness of their femininity, together with overwhelming difficulties in their interpersonal relationships, which is the usual reason for their initial referral.

Patterns of eating in bulimia vary. The patient divides her days into 'good' and 'bad' days, perhaps with deeper psychological meaning. Superficially, a good day is one when she restricts her carbohydrate and calorific intake while a bad day indicates a tendency to eat carbohydrate specifically, whether or not bulimia actually occurs. Unlike the anorectic, she enjoys food prepared by others; she finds safety from her bulimia in numbers.

Bulimia is a private affair. The patient usually has a 'safe' place where she 'allows' herself to gorge; often this is a specific room within her home where discovery of her 'illicit' pursuit is unlikely. She will lock herself in her room, take the telephone off the receiver and ignore visitors. Where the bulimia is known, attempts by friends to interrupt an attack may lead to marked anger or even overt aggression. This difficulty in stopping the bulimia, once begun, leads some boyfriends or husbands to join in or actively plan their own eating around the behaviour. Sometimes flatmates collude, perhaps vicariously.

Prior to the bulimic attack, the patient has a feeling of expectancy, elation or excitement associated with a compulsion to 'stuff' something in her mouth. The ingestion of the food is felt as humiliating, even degrading in some, although the majority describe a sense of guilt which can only be expunged by vomiting. All describe being 'bloated' and, interestingly, construe the feeling as a psychological emotion rather than a physical appreciation. The bulimia varies in frequency, the bouts becoming more frequent or more violent when the patient is emotionally stressed by interpersonal conflict. Patients find the early evening or mid-afternoon to be the most likely times when food abuse occurs. Their descriptions imply being passive victims rather than active participants in the behaviour.

Although bulimia, in the absence of psychogenic vomiting, is not uncommon, vomiting rarely occurs except after a binge. Sometimes, however, vomiting will occur after normal eating ('a bad day!') only being quiescent when the patient is actively 'dieting'. Vomiting is primarily done to remove the bloated feeling. However, emotionally it is associated with a feeling of reassurance and a determination never to binge again; it seems to have a cleansing aspect to it.

Initially, vomiting is achieved by irritating the back of the throat or by the use of a household emetic. It is not accompanied by nausea. Sometimes a more bizarre method is employed, such as presenting, bloated with food, to a casualty department, and after claiming erroneously to have taken an overdose, to have the food passively 'washed out'. Later, such methods need no longer be employed. By standing with head over a lavatory bowl, the patient can spontaneously induce a violent contraction of diaphragm and abdominal muscles to empty her stomach contents. Rarely, a patient will collect the vomit and then reingest it.

Unlike the anorectic, the bulimic patient retains enough food to maintain her body weight; breakdown of tissue fat with 'starvation ketosis' does not occur. However, there can be electrolyte disturbances, particularly so if the patient is also abusing laxatives and diuretics. Although complicated and profound disorders can result, more usually the patient appears pale and sweaty after a binge. She feels 'jittery' and may appear clinically tremulous. Fitting (see below) and tetany can occur and spikes of temperature, associated with the bulimia, preceding such symptomatology, can lead to misdiagnosis. The reason for the transient pyrexia is not known, but is perhaps related to close juxtaposition of temperature and sensitory 'centres' in the hypothalamus.

Laxative and diuretic abuse do not seem to be as emotionally laden as psychogenic vomiting. They are comparatively more easy to give up. However, vast numbers of the tablets can be taken. Rarely does the general practitioner prescribe enough diuretics, so the patient resorts to an illicit supply or gets them from a 'private' doctor.

In a recent study by the author (Lacey, 1980) of 20 patients fulfilling the criteria of the bulimic syndrome, the most common associated symptoms were menstrual irregularities and purgative abuse (Table 9.1). All the patients either purged or vomited in association with their bulimia.

Twelve (60%) of the sample described amenorrhoea of at least 10 months' duration (Table 9.2). One subject had no menstrual bleeding, despite being on the contraceptive pill. A further four subjects described irregular menstruation and three more described regular bleeds – these were all on the contraceptive pill. Only one subject had a

Table 9.1 *Declared symptoms of 20 consecutive clinic patients*

Symptom	*Patients affected*
Bulimia	20
Vomiting	15
Purging	17
Diuretic abuse	4
Menstrual dysfunction	16–19

Table 9.2 *Menstrual activity of 20 consecutive clinic patients*

	Patients affected	*On 'pill'*
Amenorrhoea	12	1
Irregular menstruation	4	1
Regular 'bleeds'	3	3
Normal menstruation	1	0

normal menstrual cycle and was not on the contraceptive pill.

That there should be such a profound disorder of menstrual function in women at *normal* body weight is intriguing, and supports the clinical finding that amenorrhoea in anorexia nervosa occurs very early in the condition before profound weight loss, and that maybe the symptom is related to factors other than just weight loss. Menstrual irregularities are also common in gross obesity. All these groups manipulate, or more rarely avoid, carbohydrate foods. The author would postulate that the most likely cause of menstrual irregularity in all the dietary disorder groups is their gross carbohydrate manipulation. This adds support to the finding (see above) that carbohydrate variation is associated with menstrual activity in normal schoolgirls. Underfed populations living in the third world are starved particularly of proteins and fats, their energy intake deriving mainly from carbohydrates. Such people maintain their birth rates, irrespective of the degree of starvation, again suggestive of the hypothesis that a supply of carbohydrates will maintain menstruation.

The patients in the sample tended to come from social classes I, II and III (Table 9.3). This is a similar distribution to that observed in anorexia nervosa studies.

However, interestingly, the social class pattern of the fathers of the patients is markedly dissimilar to that of their daughters. A total of fourteen fathers (70%) came from social classes IV and V. It is quite clear that dietary chaotics tend to move social class during their adolescent years, mainly due to education. They feel estranged and isolated from their background.

The patients tend to fall into three major groups: neurotic, personality disorder, and epileptiform.

Table 9.3 *Social class pattern of 20 female bulimics and their fathers*

Social class	*Patients*	*Fathers of patients*
I Professional	1	0
II Intermediate	12	1
III Skilled	6	5
IV Semi-skilled	1	12
V Unskilled	0	2
Total	20	20

NEUROTIC GROUP

This is the largest group and there are two main clinical presentations. The predominant clinical symptom, apart from the eating disorder, is depression or sadness. Frequently, such patients have been previously diagnosed as 'reactive depressives' and there is usually a history of overdosing. The patients tend to be quiet, shy women declaring sadness but denying the profound anger which more exactly describes their feelings. A smaller number present with anxiety-phobic features. Such patients may describe their eating behaviour in depersonalized terms; it is as if they observe their bulimic behaviour as an automaton from afar, their bodies being divorced from themselves. Again, there is a barely hidden, yet undeclared anger, which is free-floating but may be directed towards the patient herself or more usually a male partner. The abnormal eating behaviour usually starts within the context of the failure of the patient's first major sexual relationship, or following a series of brief, but abortive, relationships. The patient, wounded, critically examines herself and feels a marked low self-esteem. She feels a failure as a woman and projects this failure on to her body shape. By dieting and altering her shape she feels she can alter herself, but quickly stumbles into bulimia, a symptom which reinforces her sense of failure. Sometimes the bulimia begins during pregnancy or in the puerperium. In such cases the psychogenic vomiting is a continuation of morning sickness. Again, the pattern of eating behaviour is associated with the feeling of being a failure; usually such patients doubt their maternal feelings and find themselves struggling and depressed in caring for their new infant. In all cases, the patient seems to be struggling to achieve a perfect yet stereotyped feminine role.

The trigger of their dietary chaos is complicated, but the emotional turmoil of late adolescence and movement of social class by education are persistent features. Attempting to identify with the *slimmer* body shape and *lower* body weight of their middle-class schoolgirl peers, they begin to relate social and emotional security with carbohydrate abstention. 'Dieting', or more accurately, carbohydrate avoidance, is seen as a means of bringing control to the chaos they feel in and around their lives. They link their body shape (and weight) emotionally and socially, and to their sexuality, a matter about which these patients are so unsure that their body shape and its manipulation becomes all-enveloping. Logically, as they see it, the manipulation of shape and weight becomes the answer to *any* major emotional stress. The syndrome seems to be a clear extension to the compulsive eating common in late adolescent middle-class girls referred to above.

PERSONALITY DISORDER GROUP

Clinically, this is a much smaller group. Such patients tend to be emotionally shallow and affectively immature. The intensity varies from the dramatic somewhat histrionic personality to the frankly psychopathic. Manipulation of food is associated, to varying degrees, with alcohol and drug abuse. The patients tend to see food in a similar light to alcohol and psychotrophic drugs. They 'use' them interchangeably and in a similar way. They thus binge with alcohol and describe alterations of brief bouts of grossly pathological drinking with long phases of normality during which they are able to drink socially or to abstain altogether. Phases of drinking, like their bulimia, may commence with explosive suddenness. Similar behaviour is shown to the addictive drugs, the choice of drug depending more on their current acquaintances than personal choice.

The same impulsive out-of-control behaviour can extend to the sexual sphere with periods of sexual disinhibition. Many patients frankly describe this as 'promiscuity'. Others avoid sexual activity, but admit to a frank fear of 'going out of control' which leads them to 'safe' relationships. The hallmark of such relationships is the lack of commitment and demand within them, though there is usually an overriding affection. The men may be married and unprepared or unable to make a commitment to the patient. Others may be homosexual or bisexual, yet others are described as 'weak'. The patient finds the lack of meaning or long-term commitment within the relationship reassuring, safe and uncomplicated, her own doubts being dealt with by humiliation of her more passive partner. The humiliation or devaluation of the sexual partner seems to be a part of a desperate attempt to deny feelings of dependence. So interrelated is bulimia and sexual activity in the minds of such patients that they may use intercourse or masturbation as a means of thwarting a bulimic attack, or, alternatively, gorging to sedation may be used to lower heightened sexual drive. Fellatio may be the sole and exclusive form of sexual relationship.

Although the more histrionic patient commonly describes incestuous fantasy and often relates this to her father's difficulty at accepting her pubertal development, this has rarely led to overt sexual activity between them. Occasional homosexual relationships are described, and a similar lack of feeling that marks the patient's heterosexual relationships is noteworthy. Homosexuality tends to be used as a protection, a way of seeking sexual release without meaningful commitment or future. It rarely indicates a true homosexual orientation. Temporary and brief prostitution is resorted to by a small number.

Bulimia becomes pronounced when the patient tires of her protective but weak relationship and feels tempted into another; alternatively, dissatisfaction with the barrenness of her relationship leads to attempts to seek meaning by lowering her emotional defences. Fear, however, soon leads to her seeking solace in marked bulimia. A married lover may become divorced, a bisexual partner may move on to greener pastures, a husband may be just too inadequate; whatever the stimulus, the implications are the same and gorging the result.

In summary, such patients declare marked unsureness of their femininity and sexuality, together with overwhelming difficulties in interpersonal relationships which may include sexual disinhibition or a profound fear of it. Central to the disorder is a need to avoid dependence either by humiliation of themselves or their partners. These feelings are related, both temporally and psychodynamically, by the patient herself to the eating symptoms which first led her to seek help.

EPILEPTIFORM GROUP

This is the third and smallest group of patients presenting with the bulimic syndrome. Such patients describe epileptifom fits or 'absences' which predate the eating disorder. Some patients have diagnosable epilepsy, but more show epileptiform phenomena on the EEG, which could be related to the impulsive feelings such patients have, these being manifest in the eating behaviour. Occasional fits can occur as a result of electrolytic abnormality, secondary to vomiting and laxative abuse. A patient showing this feature should not be placed in this category. Rather, diagnosis needs to be based on a clear history of fitting predating the bulimia or psychogenic vomiting, or the presence of epileptiform phenomena following resolution of the abnormal dietary behaviour. A constant feature in the history of these patients is that the first epileptic fit took place within the context of puberty, the insecurities of that time being heightened by the lack of control exemplified by the epileptic fit.

Numerous treatment approaches have been attempted with bulimic patients. Treatment varies from the use of anticonvulsants and antidepressants to behavioural and psychodynamic therapy. Reported treatment response is variable (Boskind-Lodahl, 1976; Dally and Gomez, 1979; Palmer, 1979; Russell, 1979) which is perhaps unsurprising as the clinical groups and intensity of their symptomatology are not totally comparable.

OTHER BULIMIC SYNDROMES

Anorexia nervosa has little to do with anorexia! It is, therefore, not surprising that anorectics are ravenous for food and that some, unable to avoid food any longer, eat compulsively. Anorexia nervosa patients declare a phobia of normal body weight (Crisp, 1967, Lacey, 1976) while being at a low body weight and actively avoiding, usually by avoiding food, restoration to a normal range of body weight. There are, however, a number of diagnostic differences between the major clinicians who have studied the disorder; thus, direct comparisons as to the frequency of compulsive eating within anorexia nervosa can be difficult. Halmi (1974) declared that 10% of the 94 patients in his sample were bulimic. Theander (1970) felt that 16% of his anorectics became compulsive eaters. Other writers felt that the behaviour was more common. Thus, Bruch (1974, 1976) felt that one-fifth of her patients had this problem whilst Crisp (1967) described it in a third of his research group. Other researchers with a special anorexia nervosa clinic (Beaumont, George and Smart, 1976) found a similar proportion of bulimics (25%) amongst their patients. Many clinicians have commented that bulimia and psychogenic vomiting are functions of chronicity in anorexia nervosa and, as research clinics tend to have the more persistent patients referred to them, it can be assumed that more general outpatient clinics would find the incidence of these symptoms much less.

Within the natural history of anorexia nervosa bulimia is found in three situations. Firstly, it occurs at low body weight. Such patients describe losing control of their power of abstention and maintaining their low body weight by psychogenic vomiting or purging. This symptom pattern is a progression from the strict dieting of primary anorexia nervosa. Dally and Gomez (1979) claim that this change in eating pattern occurs about 9 months after the onset of dieting in susceptible patients. Such patients are more active and more extrovert than their abstaining peers. They lack lanugo hair, tend not to have the early-morning waking which characterizes the classical anorexia nervosa syndrome (Lacey, 1976) but have severe dental problems (Hurst, Lacey and Crisp, 1977). Secondly, bulimia can occur in recovered anorectics at normal body weight. Psychogenic vomiting is not so allied to bulimia in such a group and there is a tendency for the patient to become mildly obese. Thirdly, compulsive eating with obesity is not infrequent following those anorectics who have received a prefrontal leucotomy.

It was Stunkard (1959) who described compulsive eating in patients with massive obesity. However, then it was relatively uncommon, occurring in only 8% of his sample. In common with other groups with an eating disorder, female subjects predominated, although the proportion was lower than the proportion of females in anorexia nervosa (Wardle and Beinart, 1981). Further, self-induced vomiting is rarely mentioned, which presumably explains the massive obesity. The general clinical consensus is that such patients are emotionally disturbed, and that their compulsive overeating is triggered by emotional stress. This is not substantiated by the epidemiological literature (Crisp *et al.*, 1980;

Moore, Stunkard and Srole, 1962) which suggests that there are marked differences between mild obesity and massive obesity, and between obesity in general populations and those obese patients who present themselves to obesity clinics. It is suggested that there are lower levels of neurotic symptomatology in patients who are mildly overweight, compared with normal weight populations.

CONCLUSION

Compulsive eating seems to be a fairly common behaviour, particularly among young women. By no means is the symptom restricted to massive obesity of anorexia nervosa. It is widespread amongst general populations, although the degree of distress caused by the symptom is unknown. However, it can become in extreme cases the focus of a neurotic syndrome occurring at normal body weight. This bulimic syndrome is separated by definition from anorexia nervosa and massive obesity and, by degree, from the mild, periodic overeating which seems so common in general female populations. Although a heterogeneous disorder, the bulimic syndrome appears to have a distinct clinical presentation and aetiology. Both the symptom and the syndrome seem to have their roots in psychological, social and biological concepts of sexuality.

REFERENCES

Beaumont, P. J. V., George, G. C. W. and Smart, D. E. (1976). 'Dieters' and 'vomiters and purgers' in anorexia nervosa. *Psychol. Med.* **6**, 617

Boskind-Lodahl, M. (1976). Cinderella's stepsisters: a feminist perspective on anorexia nervosa and bulimia. *Signs*, **2**, 342

Bruch, H. (1974). *Eating Disorders.* (London: Routledge and Kegan Paul)

Bruch, H. (1976). The treatment of eating disorders. *Mayo Clin. Proc.*, **51**, 266

Crisp, A. H. (1967). The possible significance of some behavioural correlates of weight and carbohydrate intake. *J. Psychosom. Res.*, **2**, 117

Crisp, A. H. and Kalucy, R. S. (1974). Aspects of the perceptual disorder in anorexia nervosa. *Br. J. Med. Psychol.*, **1**, **47**, 349

Crisp, A. H., Queenan, M., Sittampaln, Y. and Harris, G. (1980). Jolly fat revisited. *J. Psychosom. Res.*, **24**, 233

Dally, P. and Gomez, J. (1979). *Anorexia Nervosa.* London: William Heinemann Medical Books

Feighner, J. P. (1972). Diagnostic criteria for use in psychiatric research. *Arch. Gen. Psychiatry*, **26**, 57

Frisch, R. E. and McArthur, J. W. (1974). Menstrual cycles: fatness as a determinant of minimum weight for height necessary for their maintenance or onset. *Science*, **185**, 949

Gardner, D. M. and Garfinkel, P. E. (1980). Sociocultural factors in the development of anorexia nervosa. *Psychol. Med.*, **9**, 605

Halmi, K. A. (1973). Anorexia nervosa: demographic and clinical features in 94 cases. *Psychosom. Med.*, **3**, 521

Huenemann, R. L., Shapiro, L. R., Hampton, M. C. and Mitchell, B. W. (1966). A longitudinal study of gross body composition and body conformation and their association with food and activity in a teenage population. *Am. J. Clin. Nutr.*, **18**, 325

Hurst, P. S., Lacey, J. H. and Crisp, A. H. (1977). Teeth, vomiting and diet: a study of the dental characteristics of seventeen anorexia nervosa patients. *Postgrad. Med. J.*, **53**, 298

Lacey, J. H. (1975). Anorexia nervosa. *Nursing Times*, 72, **11**, 407

Lacey, J. H. (1980). Dietary chaos – a compulsive eating syndrome. *Proceedings 13th European Conference of Psychosomatic Research, Istanbul*

Lacey, J. H., Chadbund, C., Crisp, A. H., Whitehead, J. and Stordy, J. (1978). Variation in energy intake of adolescent girls. *J. Human Nutr.*, **32**, 419

Lacey, J. H., Crisp, A. H., Kalucy, R. S., Hartmann, M. K. and Chen, C. N. (1973). Weight gain and the sleeping electroencephalogram: study of 10 patients with anorexia nervosa. *Br. Med. J.*, **2**, 556

Moore, M. D., Stunkard, A. and Srole, L. (1962). Obesity, social class and mental illness. *J. Am. Med. Assoc.*, **181**, 962

Nylander, I. (1971). The feeling of being fat and dieting in a school population. *Acta Sociol. Med. Scand.*, **1**, 17

Palmer, R. L. (1979). The dietary chaos syndrome: a useful new term? *Br. J. Med. Psychol.*, **52**, 187

Palmer, R. L., Crisp, A. H., MacKinnon, P. C. B., Franklin, M., Bonnar, J. and Wheeler, M. (1975). Pituitary sensitivity to 50 μg LH/FSH-RH in subjects with anorexia nervosa in acute and recovery stages. *Br. Med. J.*, **1**, 179

Russell, G. F. M. (1970). Anorexia nervosa: Its identity as an illness and its treatment. In J. H. Price (ed.). *Modern Trends in Psychological Medicine, II.* (New York: Appleton-Century-Crofts)

Russell, G. F. M. (1979). Bulimia nervosa: an ominous variant of anorexia nervosa. *Psychol. Med.*, **9**, 429

Stunkard, A. J. (1959). Eating patterns and obesity. *Psychiatr. Q.*, **33**, 284

Theander, S. (1970). Anorexia nervosa: a psychiatric investigation of 94 female patients. *Acta Psychiatr. Scand.*, **Suppl. 214**

Vandereycken, W. and Pierloot, R. (1980). Dysorexia: bulimia and anorexia nervosa. *Proceedings 13th European Conference on Psychosomatic Research, Istanbul*

Wardle, J. and Beinart, H. (1981). Binge eating: a theoretical review. *Br. J. Clin. Psychol.*

Ziolko, H. U. (1976). Hyperorexia nervosa. *Psychother. Med. Psychol.*, **26**, 10

Index